Dental Trauma
at a Glance

Dental Trauma at a Glance

Aws Alani
BDS, MFDS, MSc, FDS, LLM, MFDT
Specialist in Restorative Dentistry, Endodontics and Prosthodontics
London, UK

Gareth Calvert
BDS (Glas), MRes, MFDS, FDS Rest Dent RCPS (Glas)
Consultant in Restorative Dentistry and Honorary Clinical Senior Lecturer
Glasgow Dental Hospital and School
Glasgow, UK

WILEY Blackwell

Registered Offices
John Wiley & Sons, Inc., 111 River Street, Hoboken, NJ 07030, USA
John Wiley & Sons Ltd, The Atrium, Southern Gate, Chichester, West Sussex, PO19 8SQ, UK

Editorial Office
9600 Garsington Road, Oxford, OX4 2DQ, UK

For details of our global editorial offices, customer services, and more information about Wiley products visit us at www.wiley.com.

Wiley also publishes its books in a variety of electronic formats and by print-on-demand. Some content that appears in standard print versions of this book may not be available in other formats.

Library of Congress Cataloging-in-Publication Data

Names: Alani, Aws, 1979– author. | Calvert, Gareth, 1985– author.
Title: Dental trauma at a glance / Aws Alani, Gareth Calvert.
Other titles: At a glance series (Oxford, England)
Description: First edition. | Hoboken, NJ : Wiley-Blackwell, 2021. |
    Series: At a glance series | Includes bibliographical references and index.
Identifiers: LCCN 2020032912 (print) | LCCN 2020032913 (ebook) | ISBN
    9781119562832 (paperback) | ISBN 9781119563013 (adobe pdf) | ISBN
    9781119562993 (epub)
Subjects: MESH: Oral Surgical Procedures–methods | Tooth Injuries–surgery
    Tooth avulsion | Tooth luxation | Tooth fracture | Pulpotomy |
    Wounds and Injuries–surgery | Handbook
Classification: LCC RK490 (print) | LCC RK490 (ebook) | NLM WU 49 | DDC
    617.6044–dc23
LC record available at https://lccn.loc.gov/2020032912
LC ebook record available at https://lccn.loc.gov/2020032913

Cover Design: Wiley
Cover Image: ©Courtesy of Gareth Calvert and Aws Alani

Set in 9.5/11.5pt Minion by SPi Global, Pondicherry, India

Printed in Singapore
M095271_130421

Aws and Gareth wish to thank their families for their love and support, and their colleagues who inspire and motivate them.

Contents

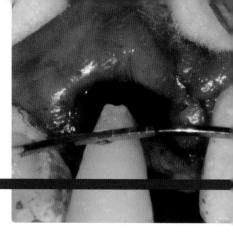

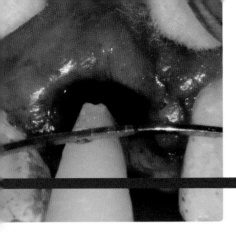

Foreword

Dental trauma is a core topic in both undergraduate and postgraduate education within Endodontology. As a consequence, there is a clear need for books that summarise the contemporary scientific evidence as well as the best clinical practice in a format that is understandable and easy to follow. This new book, *Dental Trauma at a Glance*, fulfils that need and is a timely addition to the literature and an excellent resource for those searching for information.

Traumatic dental injuries are unplanned, and they create unique challenges for dentists and other health care practitioners. *Dental Trauma at a Glance* provides all the information required to manage such injuries. The chapters in the book are logically arranged to mirror a patient journey, and the intuitive layout of each chapter walks the reader through the management of all forms of adult dental trauma.

The authors of this textbook have gone to great lengths to illustrate every chapter with real clinical examples and clear illustrations. The identical format of each chapter aids readability and allows problem-solving when traumatic dental injuries present in a step-by-step logical process.

Two specific chapters worth mentioning are 'Features of luxation injuries and principles of repositioning' as well as 'Follow-up and splint removal.' The authors firmly believe there is a right way and wrong way to do everything, and when the pressure of unfamiliar acute dental trauma becomes all the more real, these critical chapters will ensure the best clinical practice can be followed.

The simplicity of the book transcends all clinical backgrounds, from undergraduate to specialist. In the words of Einstein – 'if you can't explain it simply, you don't understand it well enough.'

Paul MH Dummer
Emeritus Professor

Preface

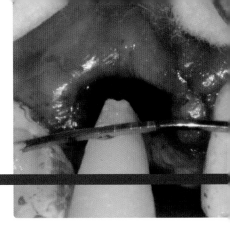

We live in a world where accidents, mishaps, disagreements, and unfortunate altercations occur on a daily basis. Both Gareth and myself have lived and worked in a variety of huge, busy cities around the United Kingdom, where dental trauma occurs under a variety of circumstances and situations. Such is the burden on health care professionals and services we were motivated to create a text that is quick to refer to and easy to understand in the hope that the scope of management of these cases is shared far and wide.

No two dental trauma cases are the same, and no story charting the circumstances of the injury cease to intrigue or cause dismay. My first memory of managing an acute traumatic injury was in South Wales as a junior trainee. A young boy had challenged his friend to shoot an apple off the top of his head 'Robin Hood' style. . .with an air rifle! Unfortunately, the apple escaped unscathed, but his central incisor was shattered. What was more apparent than the injury itself was the mental anguish on his face at the thought of a near-death experience and, of course, the appearance of his tooth. It was safe to say his mother was also as equally mortified. What we both have realised through our daily experiences is the mental trauma that dental injuries can cause our patients. Post-traumatic stress disorder is a real and significant consideration for this patient cohort, and this is an aspect of our care we must not overlook or fail to recognise. Indeed quick, efficient, and TIMELY management of dental trauma is likely to reduce the mental anguish and significant comorbidities that may develop in the future. We both feel that the complications that arise from trauma injuries are significantly more difficult and complicated to attend to than if the injury was managed optimally in the first instance. The legacy of poorly managed trauma is long and unrelenting.

We have known each other for over a decade now, worked together on numerous projects and travelled the world from Ghana to Las Vegas. I must say this book is a testament of a true friendship by two clinicians who want to make a difference for dental trauma patients around the world.

Aws Alani

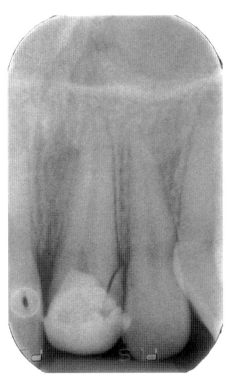

The 'shattered' central incisor

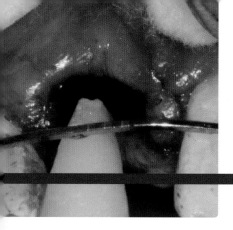

About the companion website

Don't forget to visit the companion website for this book:

www.wiley.com/go/alani/dental_trauma

There you will find valuable materials, including:

- Figures from within the book
- MCQs

Scan this QR code to visit the companion website:

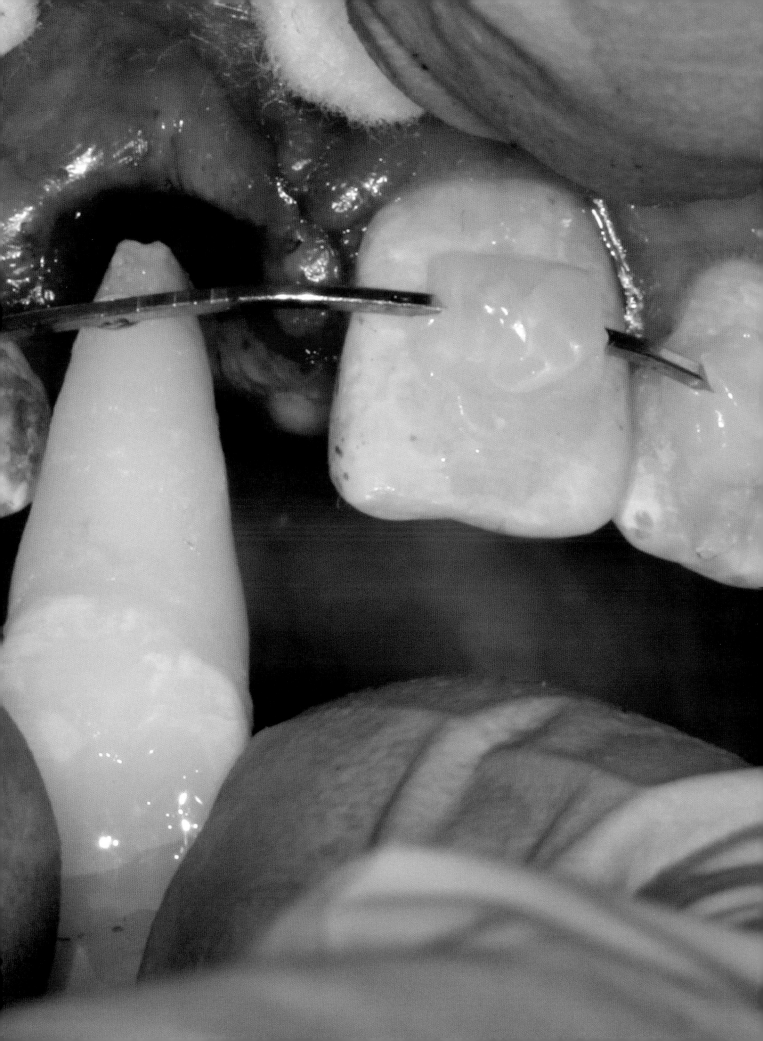

1 Risk factors for dental trauma

Figure 1.1 Demonstration of a 6mm overjet.

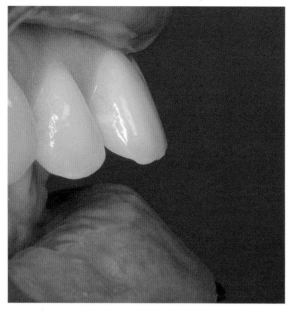

Figure 1.2 Lower lip trapped behind the maxillary incisor.

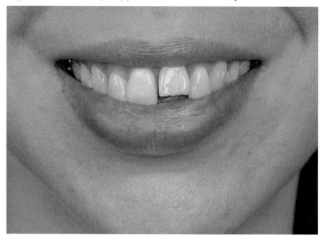

Figure 1.3 A heavily restored dentition following dental trauma with numerous fractured and decemented restorations.

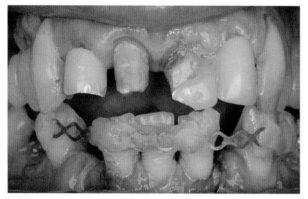

Figure 1.4 Dental trauma caused by sporting activities, in this case boxing.

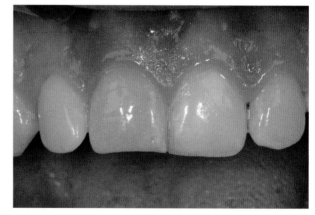

Figure 1.5 Dental trauma caused by a road traffic accident presenting 2 years later with severe hard and soft tissue defects.

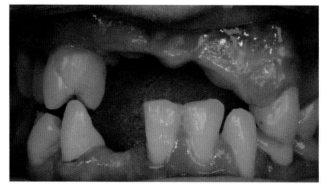

Dental Trauma at a Glance, First Edition. Aws Alani and Gareth Calvert. © 2021 John Wiley & Sons Ltd. Published 2021 by John Wiley & Sons Ltd.
Companion website: www.wiley.com/go/alani/dental_trauma

Introduction

With any acquired defects or injuries, the basis for management is the identification of risk factors and their reduction to maximise preventative strategies. By instigating awareness amongst the public, injuries can be avoided, and the burden of their management during the patient's life can be mitigated or completely removed. At worst, the severity of injuries can be reduced, making them easier to manage and resolve. Dental trauma injuries such as avulsion or intrusion can be complicated and challenging for the clinician, whereas conditions that involve luxation type injuries are easier to plan and manage future physiological or biological changes during the lifetime of the patient. The following are common risk factors (Glendor 2009).

Oral predisposing factors

- Patients with an overjet of 6 mm or greater (Figure 1.1).
- Lip incompetence (Figure 1.2).
- Protruding upper anterior teeth.
- Patients with residual dental disease, such as heavily restored teeth or periodontitis, are more likely to suffer greater consequences of trauma than those with otherwise intact healthy dentitions (Figure 1.3).

Unintentional traumatic dental injuries

- Formulates a large cohort of dental injuries.
- Patients prone to falling over due to medical conditions or those that may be at a greater risk due to seizures such as epilepsy may present multiple times throughout their lives.
- Sports that involve projectile equipment such as hockey, cricket, or football are also at a greater risk. Ice hockey has been shown to have the highest prevalence of all sports.
- Contact sports such as boxing and martial arts also carry an increased risk.
- Non-contact sports such as gymnastics, horse riding, and athletics also represent a risk.

Socioeconomic factors

- There is some evidence that shows areas with greater deprivation have a higher prevalence of trauma.
- Densely populated areas also show a greater prevalence.

Human behaviour

- Patients who take risks with their physical safety are at a greater risk of dental trauma (Figure 1.4).
- Situations of greater interpersonal difficulty such as being bullied have a higher risk of dental trauma.
- Patients who are hyperactive, such as those with Attention deficit hyperactivity disorder or ADHD, are at a greater risk of dental trauma.
- Inappropriate use of teeth such as the opening of bottles or beverages also has a higher risk of dental trauma.

Learning difficulties or physical limitations

- Epilepsy, cerebral palsy, learning difficulties, or hearing or visual impairment all present a greater risk of dental trauma.

Intentional traumatic dental injuries

- Interpersonal violence such as physical abuse between partners or assault increases the risk of dental trauma.
- Clinicians must be vigilant for signs of physical abuse and consider liaising with their local safeguarding team or seeking advice from the Police.

Iatrogenic injuries

- One of the most common complications of general anaesthesia is dental trauma during intubation procedures.

Road traffic accidents

- More severe traumatic dental injuries are likely in road traffic accidents. Due to the severity of other, likely life-threatening injuries, management of dental trauma may be delayed (Figure 1.5).

KEY POINTS
- Management of risk is the key to prevention.
- Those patients who have previously suffered dental trauma are more likely to have repeated episodes of dental trauma.
- The patient's social circumstances play a huge role in the risk of trauma.
- Medical conditions affecting movement and proneness to falling also play a significant role.
- A risk assessment should be conducted for all patients to identify those that may benefit from preventive measures.

2 Prevention of dental trauma

Figure 2.1 An example of a 'boil in the bag' mouth guard.

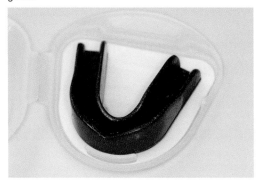

Figure 2.2 A correctly extended maxillary mouth guard covering the teeth and soft tissue following the depth of the sulcus.

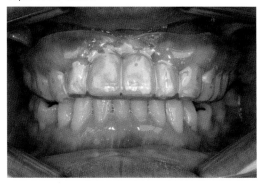

Figure 2.3 An incorrectly extended maxillary mouth guard not covering the soft tissues adequately into the sulcus leaving this area unprotected.

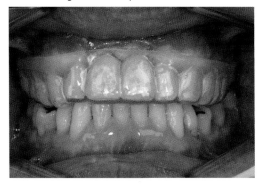

Figure 2.4 Helmets for bike travel can reduce injury severity.

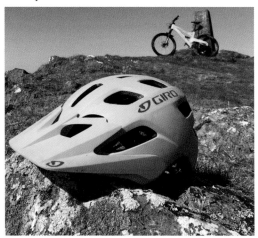

Figure 2.5 Orthodontics reducing an increased overjet.

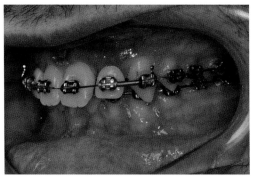

Dental Trauma at a Glance, First Edition. Aws Alani and Gareth Calvert. © 2021 John Wiley & Sons Ltd. Published 2021 by John Wiley & Sons Ltd.
Companion website: www.wiley.com/go/alani/dental_trauma

Introduction

The majority of traumatic dental injuries can happen unexpectedly during daily life. This makes their complete prevention practically impossible. Therefore education on avoidance, reduction and the correct acute management may go some way in reducing the severity of injuries, making them easier to manage once they present to the clinician.

The following are some active steps that can be taken to avoid or reduce injuries to the dental hard and soft tissues.

Mouth guards

It is recommended that all athletes wear a mouth guard or gum shield to minimise any impact and reduce the prevalence of traumatic dental injuries (Fernandes et al. 2019). The mode of protection provided by a mouth guard varies depending on the direction and energy of the impact.

There are three types of mouth guard:

- Stock (universal)
- Mouth-formed (boil and bite) (Figure 2.1)
- Custom-made (fabricated by a dental professional) (Figure 2.2)

While custom-made mouth guards from a dentist are more costly, they provide the best comfort and protection against dental trauma (Johnston and Messer 1996). Furthermore, the cost of a customised mouth guard is insignificant when compared to the financial outlay of the provision and subsequent lifelong maintenance of traumatised teeth or their prosthodontic replacement.

Ideal features of mouth guards

- Absorb and deflect frontal or axial impacts.
- Protect the oral soft tissue as well as the hard tissues (Figure 2.2).
- Support the mandible when in occlusion from crown-root fractures and mandibular jaw fracture.

Common pitfalls

- Underextension over the gingiva and mucosa (Figure 2.3). The teeth and soft tissues should be covered to increase protection, retention, and strength of the mouth guard.
- Underextension over posterior units. The mouth guard should extend over at least one molar each side for retention and occlusal stability.
- Palatal extension. The mouth guard should extend palatally in the anterior region for strength and retention.
- Thickness. If too thick, the wearer my struggle with comfort or breathing. If too thin, there will be no protective benefit.

Helmet

Wearing a helmet (Figure 2.4) or face mask for motorsports, bicycle riding, and those who use motorbikes to commute has been shown to reduce maxillofacial injuries by up to 50% (Kelly et al. 1991; Benson et al. 1999).

Unfortunately, cyclists still experience a high prevalence of dental trauma as few wear mouth guards.

Seat belts

This is a legal requirement when traveling in a motor vehicle. The use of seat belts has been shown to significantly decrease the frequency of facial injuries (Reath et al. 1989).

Overjet reduction

An increased overjet of more than 6 mm is associated with a higher prevalence of dental trauma. Therefore, orthodontic treatment to reduce the overjet should be considered in these patients (Figure 2.5).

Past experience

People with a history of dental trauma are almost three times more likely to experience another episode of dental trauma. Therefore in this cohort, these preventative measurements should be strongly considered.

KEY POINTS

- These relatively simple measures should be reinforced as they reduce the long term burden of traumatic dental injuries.

3 Essential armamentarium

Figure 3.1 Radiograph (phosphor plates) sizes for dental trauma.

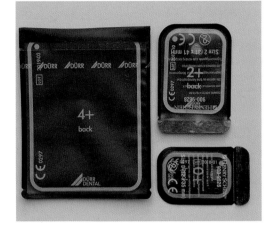

Figure 3.2 Basic equipment for repositioning and splinting traumatised teeth.

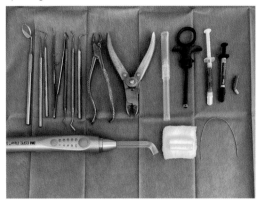

Figure 3.3 Extended range of dental equipment for splinting and endodontics.

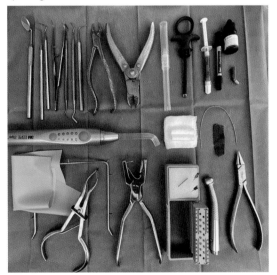

Figure 3.4 Pulp testing equipment. (a) Electric pulp test (b) Cold test.

(a)

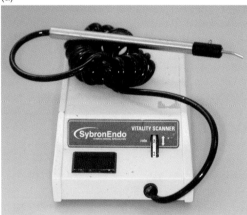

(b)

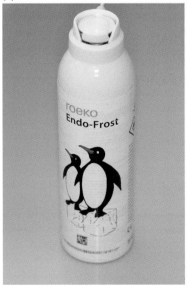

Figure 3.5 Tungsten carbide bur for removing composite during splint removal.

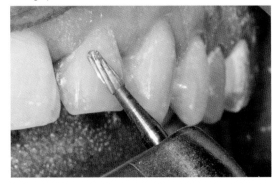

Dental Trauma at a Glance, First Edition. Aws Alani and Gareth Calvert. © 2021 John Wiley & Sons Ltd. Published 2021 by John Wiley & Sons Ltd.
Companion website: www.wiley.com/go/alani/dental_trauma

Introduction

To provide optimal treatment when acute trauma presents the clinician requires the correct equipment to be readily available. Without an organised armamentarium the clinician is less likely to be able to achieve treatment goals during the crucial period immediately post trauma (Chauhan et al. 2016).

Team approach

The importance of a team approach for the management of acute dental trauma cannot be understated:

- A family member/friend provides valuable moral support during this time of distress, and importantly another source to recall information regarding the accident itself or to ensure that post-operative instructions are followed.
- Reception staff can assist the individual in recording their personal information and medical history.
- The dental nurse is another source of reassurance for the patient during this anxious time, but most importantly, another set of hands to optimise the management of the injuries as access and dexterity in a lacerated or swollen mouth is fraught with unique challenges.

Equipment for diagnosis

- A photo of the patient's teeth prior to the trauma provides invaluable information for the clinician regarding how to reposition the teeth to their original position (such as a 'selfie' or a high-resolution portrait photo) (Djemal and Singh 2016).
- Pre-operative photographs. This will provide a plethora of information for future planning and review. A digital photo taken with a macro lens and ring flash is the optimal setup. One further important aspect may include the potential for future litigation where the injuries were non-accidental.
- Pre-operative radiographs. Size '0' '2' and, if possible, '4' films are required for periapical and occlusal radiographs, respectively (Figure 3.1). More intricate injuries and complications may only be visualised with cone beam computed tomography.

Equipment for repositioning teeth

- Almost all patients require local anaesthesia.
- Basic instrument kit (Figure 3.2).
- The majority of teeth can be repositioned using firm digital pressure. If the teeth are slippery, then a piece of gauze may aide gripping of the teeth.
- Where teeth are intruded or severely luxated, the clinician could consider the use of forceps to reposition.

Equipment for tooth stabilisation

- Once teeth have been stabilised, moisture control can take the form of either cotton rolls or cheek retraction devices.
- The most conventional method of tooth stabilisation is the passive flexible composite wire splint on the labial surfaces of the teeth.
- The splint is commonly 0.016" or 0.4mm stainless steel orthodontic wire or ribboned titanium wire.
- A wire cutter is required to cut the required length.
- Standard light cure unit (Figure 3.2).

Equipment for tooth restoration

- Where enamel or enamel and dentine fractures have occurred, the provision of a suitably contoured restoration utilising a layered composite system is advised.
- In situations where the trauma has resulted in multiple fractures and luxation injuries, making moisture control and isolation difficult, a glass ionomer cement can be utilised to stabilise prior to the more definitive restoration.

Equipment for pulp management

- Where the pulp is exposed, and the clinician identifies the need for pulpotomy or pulp capping; suitable isolation is a prerequisite, ideally with a rubber dam (Figure 3.3).
- Once isolated, a tungsten carbide bur within a fast handpiece is required to remove any inflamed tissue.
- The choice for materials to overlay the exposed pulp can vary between calcium hydroxide, mineral trioxide aggregate, or the more modern bioceramic cements.
- An intermediate layer of glass ionomer cement (GIC) underlying the definitive composite restoration will also be required.

Equipment for endodontic treatment

- Where it is envisaged that root canal treatment is inevitable, the clinician should have a basic set of instruments to extirpate and dress teeth (Figure 3.3).
- This should include the provision of rubber dam and hypochlorite irrigation in combination with calcium hydroxide dressing or other suitable dressing material.

Equipment for review and splint removal

- Cold test such as Endo-Frost™ (Coltene) (Figure 3.4), not ethyl chloride.
- Electric pulp tester (Figure 3.4).
- Once the period of splinting is completed, removal should not compromise the natural tooth tissue.

  Tungsten carbide composite removal burs in a slow handpiece provide the best outcome for this stage of treatment (Figure 3.5).

Examination of dental trauma

Figure 4.1 Extra oral examination noting (a) bilateral swelling and bruising (b) top lip laceration and abrasion.

(a)

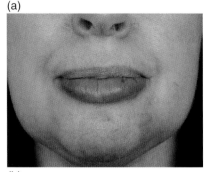

(b)

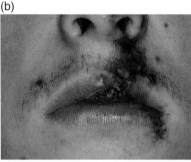

Figure 4.3 Palpation over the apex of the intruded lateral incisor would identify the step in the fractured buccal plate, clearly seen because of the fenestration through the gingiva, however may not always be as obvious.

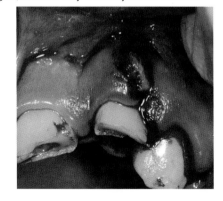

Figure 4.4 Palatally displaced maxillary incisors resulting in open bite on all remaining teeth.

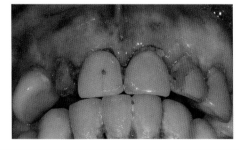

Figure 4.2 (a) Soft tissue trauma of the upper lip and palate (b) exposed bone in the midline subsequent to avulsion.

(a)

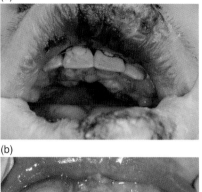

(b)

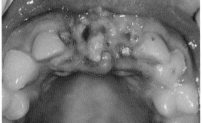

Figure 4.5 (a) Periapical radiograph of the maxillary left central incisor showing an enamel-dentine fracture repair, cervical resorption and a periapical radiolucency. (b) Maxillary occlusal radiograph of the same maxillary incisors showing hisotical trauma to adjacent teeth and the full extent of the periapical radiolucency over the lateral incisor. (c) Lateral soft tissue radiograph showing a foreign body in the upper lip and the apex of an incisor displaced labially outwith its socket consistent with a luxation injury. (d) Cone beam CT sagittal slice of a maxillary central incisor apex displaced labially with an obvious buccal alveolar plate fracture demonstrating the quintessential luxation injury.

(a)   (b)

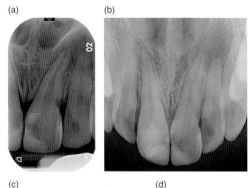

(c)   (d)

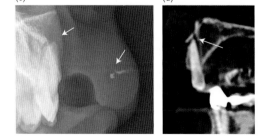

Dental Trauma at a Glance, First Edition. Aws Alani and Gareth Calvert. © 2021 John Wiley & Sons Ltd. Published 2021 by John Wiley & Sons Ltd.
Companion website: www.wiley.com/go/alani/dental_trauma

Introduction

Dental trauma is unscheduled and not frequently seen by the majority of practitioners. Therefore most are unfamiliar with its diagnosis and management.

A sound understanding of the following will avoid misdiagnosis and potentially avoidable long term complications.

Questions to ask

Was there a period of unconsciousness?

If the patient can't recall the injury, they may have lost consciousness. Enquiries should be made regarding headaches, nausea, and vomiting. If this is the case, medical attention should be sought for a head injury.

When did the injury occur?

Time is a critical factor for healing when considering treatment for avulsion and displacement injuries.

Where did the injury occur?

This could indicate a risk of contamination of the wound.

How did the injury occur?

This can indicate the region of trauma and its severity. If there are inconsistencies with the injuries and how they happened, the clinician should be suspicious of non accidental causes and be prepared for onward referral.

What emergency treatment, if any, has been carried out?

Teeth may have already been repositioned or reimplanted at the site of injury, or the patient may have come from another emergency department.

Do you have any pain or change in sensation to your skin?

This may indicate the site of injury or a disturbance in neural sensation.

Does your bite feel different?

If positive, this would suggest tooth displacement, a fracture to the jaw or temporomandibular joint.

Have you had trauma before?

Patients who experience trauma are more likely to experience a further episode of trauma. This may explain some clinical or radiographic findings.

Medical history

It is important to note immunisation history, drug allergies, blood disorders, and current medications.

Clinical examination

To allow a thorough examination, the patient's face and oral cavity usually need to be cleaned with water and gauze.

- Extraoral examination should note swellings, bruising, abrasions, and lacerations (Figure 4.1).
- Palpation of bony contours and borders of the face for steps. Flattening of the cheekbone or discomfort may indicate a fracture.
- Palpation of the soft tissue for foreign bodies (tooth fragment).
- Extent of mouth opening and any associated pain.
- Intraoral examination should note soft tissue injuries, including laceration and bruising (Figure 4.2). The latter is suggestive of a dentoalveolar fracture.
- Injuries to the hard dental tissue should then be noted – for example, missing teeth, fractured teeth, displaced teeth, or a combination of injuries. The current positioning of the teeth could be compared to a photo of the patient before their episode of dental trauma.

Clinical tests

- *Palpation* – of the bony contours may illicit a step suggestive of an underlying fracture (Figure 4.3).
- *Mobility* – increased horizontal movement of a tooth or segment of teeth is suggestive of a luxation or alveolar fracture.
- *Percussion* – will indicate periodontal ligament damage. Furthermore, a difference in tone of the percussed tooth can indicate a crushing injury, such as intrusion, or replacement resorption at a later date.
- *Occlusion* – can the patient bite together normally and comfortably (Figure 4.4).

Pulp testing

If the patient is amenable, thermal and electric testing of the pulp can be carried out. However, injured teeth can respond negatively in excess of three months before a positive response is noted (Bastos et al. 2014). Therefore it is more important to note changes in results over time.

Radiographic examination

This should focus on the area of interest highlighted by the results of the clinical examination.

Multiple angles of the adjacent and injured teeth are essential (Bourguignon et al. 2020).

What to look out for:

- Widening of the periodontal ligament (PDL) apically – this is indicative of displacement of the root tip, not periapical pathology.
- Loss of the PDL indicates intrusion.
- Interruption or change in the direction of the PDL indicates a root fracture.
- Smooth continuous outline of the alveolar housing and root form indicate no injury.

Periapical radiographs provide information on displacement injuries and cervical root and crown fractures (Figure 4.5).

Occlusal radiographs provide information on apical and middle third root fractures, alveolar fractures, and displacement injuries (Figure 4.5).

Panoramic radiographs provide information on the alveolus and facial bone fractures, including the temporomandibular joint.

Soft tissue radiographs are exposed at half the normal exposure to investigate if any tooth fragments have been retained in soft tissue lacerations (Figure 4.5).

Cone beam computed tomography (CBCT) provides a comprehensive three-dimensional view of oral and extra-oral injuries. (Figure 4.5).

Photographs

If the patient has a photograph of their teeth before the trauma, this can help inform the clinician.

Both extra- and intra-oral photographs are extremely useful for medicolegal reasons, monitoring healing, communication, and definitive treatment planning.

Signs and symptoms that warrant a referral to a maxillofacial unit

- Numbness or altered facial sensations.
- Loss or altered facial muscle control.
- Facial asymmetry or steps in facial bony contours.
- Deep lacerations or uncontrolled bleeding.
- Lack of opening.

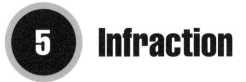

5 Infraction

Figure 5.1 Illustration of an infraction injury.

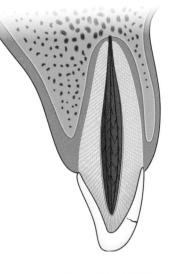

Figure 5.2 Clinical appearance of infraction or craze lines in the enamel (a) labially (b) palatally.

(a) 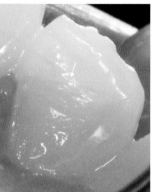 (b)

Figure 5.3 (a) Light cure illumination of an infraction injury to the maxillary right central incisor (b) tooth without light cure illumination.

(a) 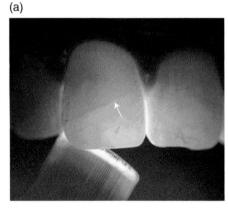 (b)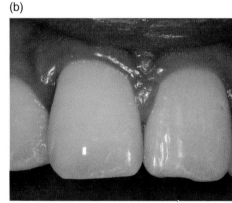

Figure 5.4 Periapical radiograph of an infraction injury.

Figure 5.5 Infraction lines with lower left lateral incisor but associated enamel fractures of the adjacent incisors.

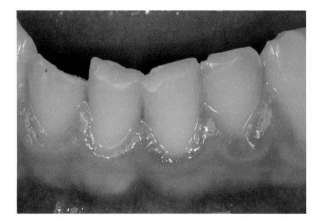

Dental Trauma at a Glance, First Edition. Aws Alani and Gareth Calvert. © 2021 John Wiley & Sons Ltd. Published 2021 by John Wiley & Sons Ltd.
Companion website: www.wiley.com/go/alani/dental_trauma

Definition

An enamel infraction is an incomplete fracture or crack running through the enamel structure parallel to the enamel rods, which stops at the dentinoenamel junction (Figure 5.1). There has usually been no loss of tooth substance.

Aetiology

Enamel infractions are caused by a direct impact to the tooth. They are most common on the labial surface of the maxillary incisors but can also be seen palatally.

Clinical examination

- Visual inspection of the crown with direct illumination will usually highlight an infraction injury. Depending on the impact, the craze lines can be seen running in various directions (Figure 5.2).
- An additional method is to use a light cure unit and illuminate the tooth from a perpendicular and parallel direction to its long axis (Figure 5.3).
- Palpation will not detect any steps in the alveolus or tenderness.
- Mobility will be normal physiological mobility.
- Percussion will not result in tenderness.
- Occlusion will be unaltered.
- There should be no evidence of periodontal damage. Otherwise, consider a concussion or subluxation injury.

Pulp test findings

A positive response can be expected from both cold and electric tests.

Radiographic findings

Periapical radiographs should show no hard tissue abnormalities (Figure 5.4).

Implications

Infractions are subtle indications of trauma and therefore, can be overlooked (Figure 5.5).

However, they can be associated with other types of injury that could be concealed subgingivally and otherwise missed.

Management

a. No splinting is required.
b. Etching and sealing with unfilled resin is recommended if the fracture lines are marked. This may prevent extrinsic staining of the fracture lines and bacterial ingress.
c. Provide post-operative instructions as advised in Chapter 21.

Follow-up

None routinely recommended.

If there are other associated injuries, follow-up is based on those injuries.

Prognosis

Pulp necrosis is very low, between 0 and 3.5%. If necrosis does occur this may be indicative of a missed concussion or luxation injury (Andreasen et al. 1985).

The periodontium is unaffected.

KEY POINTS

- Enamel infraction appears as craze lines.
- They are an indicator of a direct impact.
- Be sure there are no associated concomitant injuries of the supporting tissues.

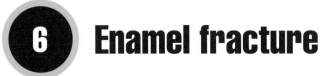

6 Enamel fracture

Figure 6.1 Illustration of an enamel fracture.

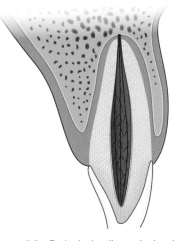

Figure 6.3 Periapical radiograph showing an enamel fracture of the (a) maxillary left central incisor and (b) mandibular left central incisor in the absence of any hard tissue injury.

(a) (b)

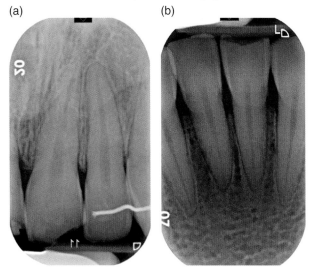

Figure 6.2 Clinical appearance of an enamel fracture of the maxillary left central incisor, note the soft tissue damage and concomitant injuries.

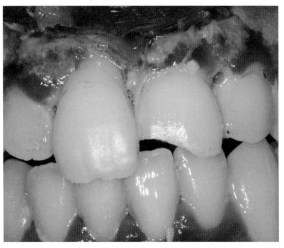

Figure 6.4 Clinical appearance of an enamel fracture of the mandibular left central incisor in conjunction with a soft tissue injury indicating an associated displacement injury.

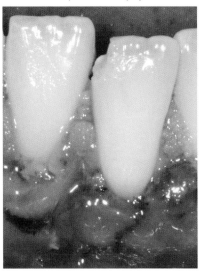

Figure 6.5 (a) Clinical appearance of a maxillary right central incisor enamel fracture (b) repaired with composite resin.

(a) (b)

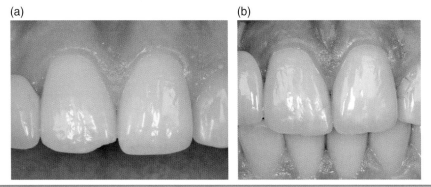

Dental Trauma at a Glance, First Edition. Aws Alani and Gareth Calvert. © 2021 John Wiley & Sons Ltd. Published 2021 by John Wiley & Sons Ltd.
Companion website: www.wiley.com/go/alani/dental_trauma

Definition

An enamel fracture is the loss of tooth substance confined to enamel only with no dentine exposure. This is also known as an uncomplicated crown fracture. (Figure 6.1).

Aetiology

Enamel fractures are caused by a direct impact of sufficient magnitude to cause loss enamel tooth structure (Andreasen 1970). This commonly includes falls, contact sports, and root traffic accidents (Gutz 1971). Crown fractures in the permanent dentition are common injuries comprising up to 76% of all dental injuries and are usually associated with maxillary central incisors (Rauschenberger and Hovland 1995).

Clinical examination

- Visual inspection of the crown will reveal the loss of enamel. No dentine will be exposed (Figure 6.2).
- Palpation will not detect any steps in the alveolus or tenderness.
- Mobility will be normal physiological mobility.
- Percussion will not result in tenderness.
- Occlusion will be unaltered.
- There should be no evidence of periodontal damage. Otherwise, consider a concussion or subluxation injury.

Pulp test findings

A positive response can be expected.

Initially, pulp testing may respond negatively. This may indicate only transient pulpal damage. Pulp testing should be repeated during follow up and only if a persistent negative response is recorded should pulp necrosis be considered in combination with the full clinical picture.

Radiographic findings

Periapical and occlusal radiographs are recommended to exclude root fracture or luxation injuries.

The enamel loss will be visible. There should be no other hard tissue abnormalities seen (Figure 6.3).

A soft tissue view could be considered if there is evidence of soft tissue lacerations.

Implications

If any clinical and radiographic findings are inconsistent, concomitant injuries to the periodontium should be suspected. This is important as luxation injuries have a negative impact on the prognosis of enamel fractures (Figure 6.4) (Andreasen et al. 1985, 1995; Lauridsen et al. 2012).

Management options

1 *If the enamel fracture is inconspicuous,* it could be smoothed with a selective enameloplasty.
2 *If the tooth fragment is available,* it can be bonded back into place:
   a. Do not chamfer the fractured surfaces; this will inhibit accurate relocation.
   b. Etch and bond each of the fractured surfaces.
   c. Do not light cure.
   d. Apply composite resin and reposition the fractured segment.
   e. Cure the composite as per manufacturer instructions. Polish any excess composite resin.
   f. If the join is visible, a chamfer margin can be created on either side of the fracture line and restored with more composite resin.
   g. Provide post-operative instructions as advised in Chapter 21.
3 *If the fragment is not available:*
   a. Immediate restoration with composite resin is advised. This can include a 1–2 mm wide chamfer preparation (Figure 6.5).
   b. Provide post-operative instructions as advised in Chapter 21.

If concomitant injuries take priority or prohibit a satisfactory restoration, the repair can be delayed.

Follow-up

Clinical pulp testing and radiographic examination are recommended at 6-8 weeks and 1 year. If there are associated luxation or root fracture injuries these follow up times should take priority.

Prognosis

Pulp necrosis is unlikely at between 0.2 and 1% (Ravn 1981).

Pulp canal obliteration and root resorption are rare findings (Stalhane and Hedegard 1975).

If the enamel fracture is associated with a luxation injury, the risk of pulpal and periodontal complications is much higher (Lauridsen et al. 2012).

KEY POINTS
- Enamel fractures do not involve dentine.
- They can be immediately restored.
- There is no need for splinting.
- Follow up at 6-8 weeks and 1 year.

7 Enamel–dentine fracture

Figure 7.1 Illustration of an enamel-dentine fracture.

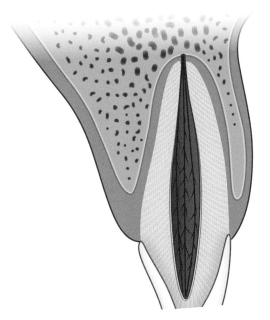

Figure 7.2 (a) Clinical appearance of an enamel-dentine fracture. (b) Note the pulp has not been breached in the occlusal view.

(a)

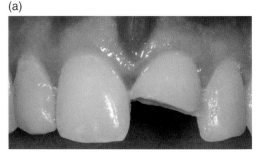

(b)

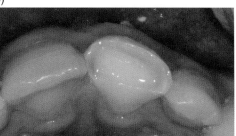

Figure 7.3 (a) Periapical and (b) occlusal radiograph showing an enamel dentine fracture provisionally repaired with glass ionomer. (c) A soft tissue radiograph showing a fragment of tooth in the lower lip.

(a)   (b)   (c)

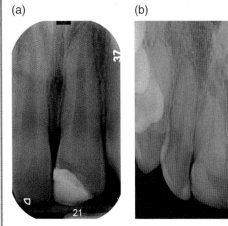

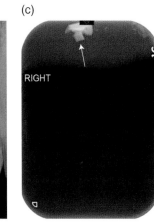

Figure 7.4 Clinical appearance of an enamel-dentine fragment retrieved from the lower lip.

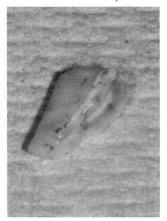

Figure 7.5 (a) Clinical appearance of a direct composite resin restoration utilising dentine and enamel layering for a fractured maxillary left central incisor. (b) the finished composite resin restoration.

(a)   (b)

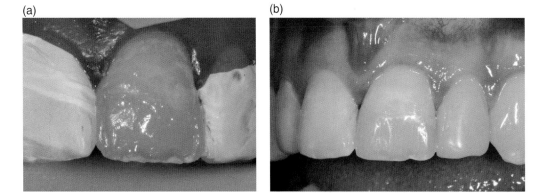

Dental Trauma at a Glance, First Edition. Aws Alani and Gareth Calvert. © 2021 John Wiley & Sons Ltd. Published 2021 by John Wiley & Sons Ltd.
Companion website: www.wiley.com/go/alani/dental_trauma

Definition

An enamel–dentine fracture is the loss of tooth substance confined to enamel and dentine (Figure 7.1). There is no pulp exposure, also known as an uncomplicated crown fracture.

Aetiology

Enamel–dentine fractures are caused by a direct impact of sufficient magnitude to cause loss of tooth structure (Andreasen 1970). This commonly includes falls, contact sports, and road traffic accidents (Gutz 1971). Crown fractures in the permanent dentition are common injuries comprising up to 76% of all dental injuries and are usually associated with maxillary central incisors (Rauschenberger and Hovland 1995).

Clinical examination

- Visual inspection of the crown will reveal loss of enamel and dentine. There will be no pulpal exposure (Figure 7.2).
- Palpation will not detect any steps in the alveolus or tenderness.
- Mobility will be normal physiological mobility.
- Percussion may result in tenderness.
- Occlusion will be unaltered.
- There should be no evidence of periodontal damage.
- If any of the above are present, be suspicious of additional concussion or luxation injuries.

Pulp test findings

Due to the exposed dentine, the patient may already complain of sensitivity to thermal changes.

A positive response to pulp testing can be expected.

However, initial pulp testing may respond negatively. This may indicate only transient pulpal damage. Pulp testing should be repeated during follow-up and only if a persistent negative response is recorded should pulp necrosis be considered in combination with the full clinical picture.

Radiographic findings

Periapical and occlusal radiographs are recommended to exclude root fracture or luxation injuries (Figure 7.3).

The loss of enamel and dentine will be visible. The remaining dentine thickness overlying the pulp should be noted.

There should be no other hard tissue abnormalities seen.

A soft tissue view could be considered if soft tissue lacerations are present to search for the tooth fragment (Figure 7.3).

Implications

Enamel–dentine crown fractures expose a large number of dentine tubules susceptible to thermal and chemical irritants and bacterial penetration, which may jeopardise the pulpal status.

If any clinical and radiographic findings are inconsistent, concomitant injuries to the periodontium should be suspected. This is important as luxation injuries have a negative impact on

the prognosis of enamel–dentine fractures (Andreasen et al. 1985, 1995; Lauridsen et al. 2012).

Management options

1 *If there are concomitant injuries* or the patient compliance precludes a satisfactory definitive restoration, the exposed dentine should be provisionally sealed with glass-ionomer.
2 *If the tooth fragment is available* (Figure 7.4), it can be bonded back into place:
   a. Do not chamfer the fractured surfaces, this will inhibit accurate relocation.
   b. Etch and bond but do not cure each of the fractured surfaces.
   c. Apply composite resin on the fractured surface and reposition the fractured segment.
   d. Cure the composite as per manufacturer instructions.
   e. Polish any excess composite resin. If the join is visible, a chamfer margin can be created on either side of the fracture line and restored with more composite resin.
   f. Provide post-operative instructions as advised in Chapter 21.
3 *If the tooth fragment is not available*:
   a. Restoration with composite resin is advised (Figure 7.5). This can include a 1–2 mm wide chamfer preparation. If there is less than 1 mm of remaining dentine thickness, an indirect pulp cap can be considered with a calcium hydroxide-based material.
   b. Provide post-operative instructions as advised in Chapter 21.

Follow-up

Clinical pulp testing and radiographic examination is recommended at 6-8 weeks and 1 year. If there are associated luxation or root fracture injuries these follow up times should take priority.

Prognosis

Bonding the fragment into position has a good medium-term survival (Andreasen et al. 1995).

Pulp necrosis is unlikely with an incidence of between 2 and 6% (Stalhane Olsburgh et al. 2002).

Pulp canal obliteration and root resorption are rare findings (Hedegard 1975).

If the enamel–dentine fracture is associated with a luxation injury, the risk of pulpal and periodontal complications is much higher (Robertson 1998).

KEY POINTS

- Enamel–dentine fractures do not involve pulp exposure.
- Exposed dentine should be immediately sealed.
- Bevelling the fractured portion should be avoided as this makes its relocation more difficult.
- Follow up at 6-8 weeks and 1 year.

8 Enamel–dentine–pulp fracture

Figure 8.1 Illustration of an enamel-dentine-pulp fracture.

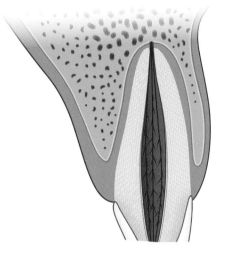

Figure 8.3 (a) Periapical radiograph showing the enamel-dentine-pulp fracture and pulpal exposure of the maxillary left canine. (b) Soft tissue radiograph confirming there is no tooth fragment contained within the lip.

(a)   (b)

Figure 8.2 (a) Clinical appearance of an enamel-dentine-pulp fracture. (b) Note the pulp exposure in the occlusal view.

(a)

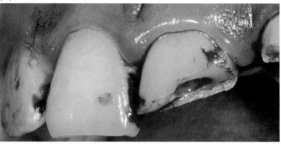

(b)

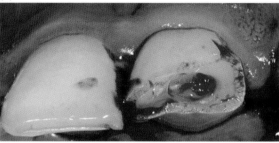

Figure 8.4 Clinical appearance of an enamel-dentine-pulp fragment.

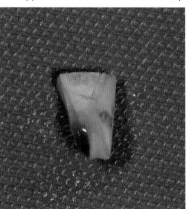

Figure 8.5 (a) Clinical appearance of an enamel-dentine-pulp (complicated) fracture of the maxillary right central incisor. (b) The pulp has been cut back by 2mm and haemostasis has been achieved. (c) The pulp has been covered with calcium hydroxide. (d) Glass ionomer cement is then overlayed prior to utilising composite resin to restore the class IV fracture. Images courtesy of Dr Abs Casaus and Dr Dan Sisson.

(a)   (b)   (c)   (d)

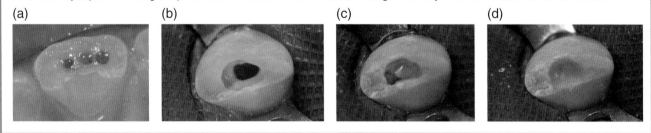

Dental Trauma at a Glance, First Edition. Aws Alani and Gareth Calvert. © 2021 John Wiley & Sons Ltd. Published 2021 by John Wiley & Sons Ltd.
Companion website: www.wiley.com/go/alani/dental_trauma

Definition

An enamel–dentine–pulp fracture involves loss of enamel and dentine tooth substance and exposure of the pulp (Figure 8.1), also known as a complicated crown fracture.

Aetiology

Complicated crown fractures are caused by a direct impact of sufficient magnitude to cause loss of tooth structure (Andreasen 1970). This commonly includes falls, contact sports, and root traffic accidents (Gutz 1971). Crown fractures in the permanent dentition are common injuries comprising up to 13% of all dental injuries and are usually associated with maxillary central incisors (Andreasen and Andreasen 1993).

Clinical examination

- Visual inspection of the crown will reveal loss of enamel, dentine, and exposure of the underlying pulp (Figure 8.2).
- Palpation will not detect any steps in the alveolus or tenderness.
- Mobility will be normal physiological mobility.
- Percussion may result in tenderness.
- There should be no evidence of periodontal damage.
- Occlusion will be unaltered.
- If any of the above are present, be suspicious of additional concussion or luxation injuries.

Pulp test findings

Due to the exposed pulp, the patient may already complain of sensitivity to thermal changes.

A positive response to pulp testing can be expected.

If pulp testing responds negatively, this may indicate only transient pulpal damage but it is a risk factor for future pulpal necrosis. Pulp testing should be repeated during follow-up and only if a persistent negative response is recorded should pulp necrosis be considered.

Radiographic findings

Periapical and occlusal radiographs are recommended to exclude root fracture or luxation injuries.

The loss of enamel, dentine, and pulp exposure will be visible (Figure 8.3). The presence of an immature apex should be noted.

There should be no other hard tissue abnormalities seen.

A soft tissue view could be considered if soft tissue lacerations are present to search for the tooth fragment (Figure 8.3).

Implications

If there is immature root development, all efforts should be made to preserve pulp vitality.

If any clinical and radiographic findings are inconsistent, concomitant injuries to the periodontium should be suspected.

Exposed pulp tissue has the capacity to heal by forming a dentine bridge. The duration of pulp exposure does not seem to have a negative effect on this mode of hard tissue healing (Cvek 1993; Olsburgh et al. 2002). Favourable healing will require an otherwise healthy pulp, intact vascular supply, exclusion of bacteria, and the use of calcium hydroxide or calcium silicate-based restorative material directly overlying the pulp.

Non-setting calcium hydroxide is the preferred material for pulpal coverage. It has a 90% success in forming a dentine barrier. In comparison utilisation of a calcium silicate cement can be technique sensitive, causes discolouration, and is relatively expensive (Bakland and Andreasen 2002).

Management

The aim is to preserve pulp vitality.

If there are extenuating circumstances that the following procedures cannot be performed in a timely manner, a bandage of resin-modified glass ionomer cement sound be applied over the fractured segment (Bakland 2009).

Otherwise:

a. Retain the tooth fragment (Figure 8.4).
b. Apply local anaesthesia.
c. Isolate the tooth with a rubber dam if there has been no associated luxation injury.
d. Clean the area with saline drenched cotton pledgets.
e. Gently disinfect the exposed enamel, dentine, and pulp with a 0.5% sodium hypochlorite soaked cotton pledget.
f. Signs that the pulp is irreversibly damaged include, contamination with debris, continuous bleeding or if it can be peeled away from the dentine walls. Therefore; take a tungsten carbide bur and with copious water spray, remove 2-3 mm of pulp.
g. Gently disinfect the area again with 0.5% sodium hypochlorite.
h. Once haemostasis is achieved, apply a thin layer of calcium hydroxide over the exposed pulp, avoid coating the adjacent dentine or enamel (Figure 8.5).
i. Restore the remaining cavity with resin-modified glass ionomer cement.
j. Apply bond on the original tooth fragment and root face; do not cure.
k. Do not chamfer the fractured surfaces as this will inhibit the relocation of the fractured portions.
l. Bond the tooth fragment in position with composite resin, or if the fragment is not available, apply direct composite resin described in Chapter 7.
m. Provide post-operative instructions as advised in Chapter 21. Due to dehydration of the tooth fragment, the colour may look different when restored. This may improve with time as the fractured portion rehydrates.

Follow-up

Clinical pulp testing and radiographic examination are recommended at 6-8, 12, 24 weeks, and one year. If there are associated luxation or root fracture injuries these follow up times should take priority.

Prognosis

Pulp necrosis and pulpal complications are rare unless associated with a concomitant luxation injury (Stalhane Olsburgh et al. 2002).

Root formation should continue.

Periodontal complications are extremely rare.

KEY POINTS

- Complicated crown fractures involve pulp exposure.
- Preserving pulp vitality is the main objective, especially if root formation is immature.
- Calcium hydroxide promotes hard tissue formation.
- Follow up at 6-8, 12, 24 weeks, and one year.

9 Crown–root fracture

Figure 9.1 Illustration of a crown-root fracture that does not involve the pulp. Note the extent of the fracture subgingivally.

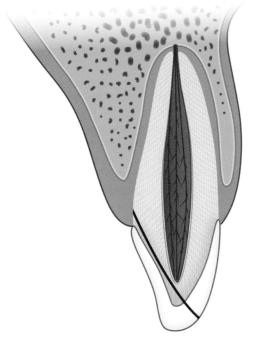

Figure 9.3 Periapical radiograph of a maxillary right central incisor with a crown-root fracture not involving the pulp. Note the apical extent of the fracture is difficult to determine.

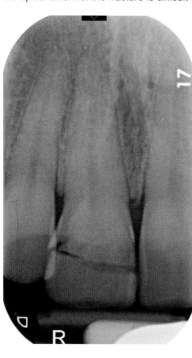

Figure 9.2 Clinical appearance of a maxillary lateral incisor with a crown-root fracture (a) from the labial aspect and (b) the occlusal aspect. Note the palatal extent of the fracture and its associated luxation injury.

(a)

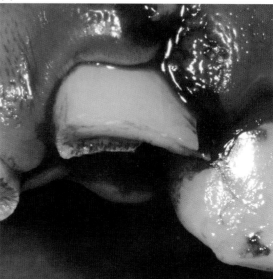

(b)

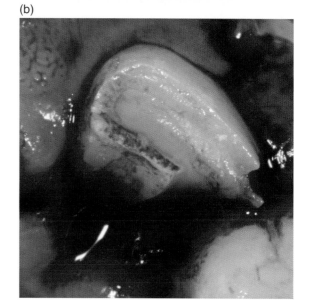

Dental Trauma at a Glance, First Edition. Aws Alani and Gareth Calvert. © 2021 John Wiley & Sons Ltd. Published 2021 by John Wiley & Sons Ltd.
Companion website: www.wiley.com/go/alani/dental_trauma

Definition

A crown–root fracture involves enamel, dentine, and cementum that extends subgingivally with loss of tooth substance. It does not involve the pulp (Figure 9.1).

Aetiology

The causes of crown–root fractures include trips, sporting accidents, road traffic accidents, and interpersonal violence (Castro et al. 2005).

Clinical examination

- The patient may present with discomfort to thermal changes.
- Visual inspection will reveal a crown fracture that extends subgingivally. The fracture usually begins supragingivally on the labial aspect and advances apically towards the palatal aspect (Figure 9.2). The coronal portion may or may not be present.
- Palpation of the tooth may be uncomfortable.
- Mobility of the coronal fragment will be noted if the fragment has not been lost.
- Percussion of the tooth will be uncomfortable for the patient.
- If retained, the fragment will be held in position by the remaining periodontal ligament attached to the coronal portion.
- Occlusal disturbance is common as the fractured coronal portion is usually displaced.

Pulp test findings

The apical fragment will usually test positive.

Pulp testing should be repeated during follow-up and only if a persistent negative response is recorded should pulp necrosis be considered in combination with the full clinical picture.

Radiographic findings

Periapical and occlusal radiographs are recommended to visualise the fracture.

A fracture will be noted, but the apical extent is usually difficult to determine (Figure 9.3). In some instances, cone beam CT imaging may be of further benefit.

Implications

The apical portion of the fractured tooth commonly maintains its neurovascular supply and vitality.

The ratio of the extent of the subgingival fracture to the length and morphology of the root is the critical factor when formulating a definitive treatment plan.

Emergency management

a. Administer local anaesthesia.
b. Wash the area with saline.
c. Splint the fractured portion as described in Chapter 20 until a definitive plan is confirmed.
d. Provide post-operative instructions as advised in Chapter 21.

Definitive treatment options

1 *Apical root portion restorable.*
2 If the fractured coronal portion is available, bond it back into position as described in Chapter 7.
3 If the fractured portion of the tooth is not available, etch bond composite resin similar to a crown fracture (see Chapter 7).
4 Alternatively restore with an indirect restoration (de Castro et al. 2010).
5 *Apical root portion restorable but requires gingivectomy or surgical crown lengthening such that asymmetrical gingiva isn't an aesthetic concern.*
6 Definitive restoration is with the fractured portion, direct composite resin, or an indirect alternative (de Castro et al. 2010).
7 *Apical root portion restorable after orthodontic extrusion.*
8 Carry out endodontic treatment and placement of a post to facilitate orthodontic extrusion. Definitive restoration with a crown (see Chapter 10) (de Castro et al. 2010).
9 *Apical root portion restorable after surgical repositioning.*
10 Splint for four weeks. Definitive restoration, as described in point 2.
11 *Apical root portion unrestorable.*
12 Decoronation to the alveolar level, leaving the root in situ to preserve bone (de Castro et al. 2010).
13 Definitive restorations include resin bonded bridgework, conventional bridgework, removable partial denture.
14 *Apical root portion unrestorable.*
15 Extraction for replacement with a single unit implant crown or conventional fixed/removable prosthodontics (de Castro et al. 2010).

Follow-up

Clinical pulp testing and radiographic examination are recommended at 1, 6-8, 12, and 24 weeks, 1 year, and annually thereafter for 5 years.

Arrange a definitive treatment planning assessment.

Prognosis at one year

There is little published evidence for pulp prognosis.

Root resorption however is more common if repositioning the tooth orthodontically or surgically (Elkhadem et al. 2014).

KEY POINTS

- The apical root portion maintains its vitality.
- The prognosis is not reduced by a short delay in definitive treatment.
- Therefore if unsure, splint the fractured portion or cover the exposed dentine and consider a second opinion on the treatment options from a specialist.
- Follow up at 1, 6-8, 12, and 24 weeks, 1 year, and annually thereafter for 5 years.

Crown–root fracture with pulp involvement

Figure 10.1 Illustration of a crown-root fracture involving the pulp.

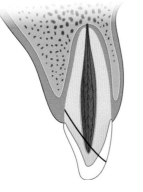

Figure 10.3 (a) Periapical radiograph of a crown-root fracture including the pulp of the maxillary left central incisor. Note the apical extent of the fracture is not immediately obvious. (b) A cone beam CT slice showing the full apical extent of the fracture.

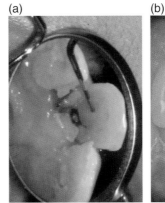

Figure 10.5 Maxillary left canine fractured tooth portion removed. In this instance the apical portion was able to be isolated with rubber dam for endodontic treatment.

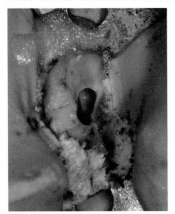

Figure 10.2 Clinical appearance of a crown-root fracture including the pulp of the maxillary left canine (a) from the labial aspect, note the fracture line running subgingivally and (b) occlusally note the pulpal exposure.

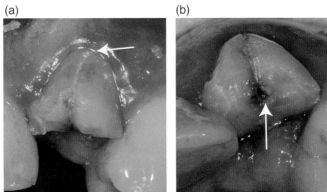

Figure 10.4 (a) A clinical example of a fracture extending palatally involving the pulp of the maxillary left central incisor. (b) splinted in position as an emergency measure before definitive treatment.

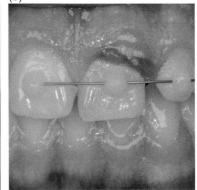

Figure 10.6 (a) Surgical crown lengthening of the maxillary left central incisor's fractured apical portion. (b) After endodontic treatment. (c) The coronal tooth portion has been bonded back in place with composite resin. Note the discolouration at the fracture line, this can be improved with a chamfer and composite resin.

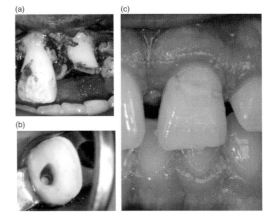

Definition

A crown–root fracture that exposes the pulp involving the enamel, dentine, cementum extending subgingivally (Figure 10.1).

Aetiology

The causes of crown–root fractures with pulp exposure include trips, sporting accidents, road traffic accidents, and interpersonal violence (Castro et al. 2005).

Clinical examination

- The patient may present with discomfort to thermal changes.
- Visual inspection will reveal a crown fracture that extends subgingivally. The fracture usually begins supragingvally on the labial aspect and advances apically on the palatal aspect. The coronal portion may or may not be present, and therefore the exposed pulp maybe visible (Figure 10.2).
- Palpation of the tooth may be uncomfortable.
- Mobility of the coronal fragment will be noted if the fragment has not been lost.
- Percussion of the tooth will be uncomfortable for the patient.
- The fragment will be held in position by the periodontal ligament attached to the fractured portion.
- Occlusal disturbance is common as the fractured coronal portion is usually displaced.

Pulp test findings

The apical fragment will usually test positive.

Pulp testing should be repeated during follow-up and only if a persistent negative response is recorded should pulp necrosis be considered in combination with the full clinical picture.

Radiographic findings

Periapical and occlusal radiographs are recommended to visualise the fracture.

A fracture will be noted, but the apical extent is usually difficult to determine (Figure 10.3). If the coronal portion is missing, the level at which the pulp is exposed will be visible. In some instances cone beam CT imaging may be of further benefit (Figure 10.3).

Implications

If there is immature root formation, preserving the pulp vitality with a pulpotomy is desirable.

The goal is to create a situation where the tooth can be confidently restored after the coronal fragment has been removed.

Emergency management

a. Administer local anaesthesia.
b. Wash the area with saline.
c. Splint the fractured tooth portion as described in Chapter 20 until a definitive plan is confirmed (Figure 10.4).
d. If the fractured tooth portion is not available, isolate the tooth and carry out a pulpotomy, as described in Chapter 8. Restore with a glass ionomer bandage.
e. Provide post-operative instructions as advised in Chapter 21.

Follow-up

Clinical pulp testing and radiographic examination are recommended at 1, 6-8, 12, 24 weeks, 1 year, and annually thereafter for 5 years.

Arrange a definitive treatment planning assessment.

Definitive treatment options

1 *If there is immature root formation and the tooth is restorable:*
  a. Perform a pulpotomy as described in Chapter 8.
  b. Then restore the tooth with either the fractured portion of the tooth, as described in Chapter 7.
  c. Or a direct composite resin described in Chapter 7.
  d. Or an indirect restoration.
    If there is complete root formation or pulpotomy is not a viable option, consider:
2 *Apical root portion restorable.*
  a. Carry out endodontic treatment. If the fractured coronal portion is available, adhesively bond it back into position.
  b. If the fractured portion is not available, restore with a definitive post-core crown.
3 *Apical root portion restorable after Orthodontic extrusion* (Figure 10.5).
  a. Carry out endodontic treatment, placement of a post to facilitate orthodontic extrusion.
  b. Restore with a definitive post-core crown.
4 *Apical root portion restorable but requires gingivectomy or surgical crown lengthening* such that asymmetrical gingiva isn't an aesthetic concern.
  a. Carry out endodontic treatment. Restore with the fractured portion or definitive post-core crown (Figure 10.6).
5 *Apical root portion restorable after surgical repositioning.*
  a. Splint for four weeks.
  b. Carry out endodontic treatment. Restore with a definitive post-core crown.
6 *Apical root portion unrestorable.*
  a. Decoronation to the alveolar level, leaving the root in situ to preserve bone.
  b. Definitive restorations include resin bonded bridgework, conventional bridgework, and removable partial denture.
7 *Apical root portion unrestorable.*
  a. Therefore extraction for replacement with a single unit implant crown or conventional fixed/removable prosthodontics.

Prognosis at one year

There is little in the way of published evidence for pulp prognosis.

Root resorption, however, is more common if repositioning the tooth orthodontically or surgically (Elkhadem et al. 2014).

KEY POINTS

- Consider pulpotomy before complete pulpectomy if there is immature root formation.
- If unsure, splint the fractured portion or cover the exposed dentine and pulp and consider a second opinion on the treatment options from a specialist.
- Follow up at 1, 6-8, 12, and 24 weeks, 1 year, and annually thereafter for 5 years.

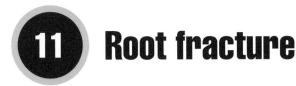

11 Root fracture

Figure 11.1 Illustration of a root fracture. This can happen at the cervical, middle and apical third of the root.

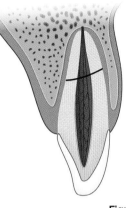

Figure 11.2 Clinical appearance of both maxillary central incisors that have middle third root fractures.

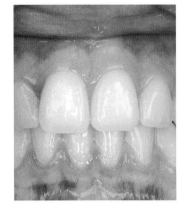

Figure 11.3 Periapical radiograph showing the middle third root fractures of both maxillary central incisors.

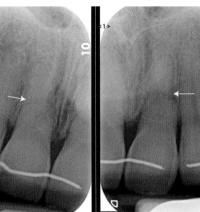

Figure 11.4 An occlusal radiograph showing the same maxillary central incisors but the true extent of the displacement between the fractured portions of root.

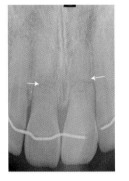

Figure 11.5 An off-centre periapical radiograph showing subtle signs of a maxillary right central incisor middle third root fracture: symmetrical lateral radiolucency in the middle root third and a step in the middle third mesial root surface.

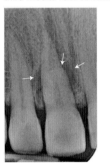

Figure 11.6 Cone beam CT image clearly showing a horizontal root fracture.

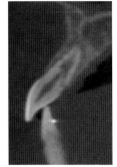

Figure 11.9 (a) This maxillary right central incisor presented with a cervical third root fracture (b) Despite the severity of the injury the tooth was maintained after splinting of up to 4 months.

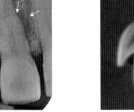

(a) (b)

Figure 11.7 Factors associated with a poor prognosis include (a) periodontal pocketing to the fracture line or a gingival fenestration, (b) displacement, bone loss and periapical radiolucency associated with the apical root fragment.

(a) (b)

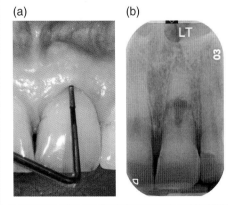

Figure 11.8 Splinting of the maxillary central incisors due to a middle root third fracture.

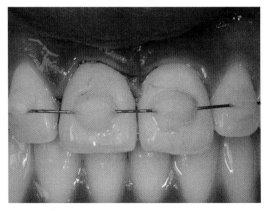

Definition

This injury is of the tooth root, which includes the cementum, dentine and pulp. Injuries can be classified into their corono-apical position, either apical, middle, or coronal third (Figure 11.1). The different classification categories is of particular importance for subsequent management and prognosis.

Aetiology

Root fractures usually occur due to a frontal impact that creates compression on the labial surface. Root fractures account for approximately 7% of all adult dental injuries. The most commonly affected tooth is the maxillary central incisor. They are commonly associated with injuries to the alveolus and soft tissue (Andreasen et al. 2004; Cvek et al. 2008; Majorana et al. 2002).

Clinical examination

- Visual inspection can reveal little (Figure 11.2). Unless the coronal fragment is displaced or there may be bleeding from the gingival sulcus.
- Palpation of the surrounding gingiva may reveal a displacement or apical tenderness.
- Mobility of the tooth may be noted if the fracture is in the coronal third.
- Percussion of the teeth may be uncomfortable for the patient.
- Occlusal disturbance will only be present if the coronal portion is displaced.

Pulp test findings

These can be inconclusive for up to three months.

Pulp testing should be repeated during follow-up and only if a persistent negative response is recorded should pulp necrosis be considered in combination with the full clinical picture.

Radiographic findings

Periapical and occlusal radiographs are recommended to visualise the fracture line.

A horizontal fracture is easily visible on a regular periapical radiograph (Figure 11.3), while an oblique fracture is more likely to be revealed on an upper standard occlusal radiograph (Figure 11.4). Radiographic signs of a root fracture can also be more subtle (Figure 11.5); therefore, in some instances, cone beam CT imaging may be of further benefit (Figure 11.6).

To differentiate between a root fracture and alveolar fracture, the alveolar fracture line will move up or down the root length according to the change in the X-ray beam angle. A root fracture will not change in position with a change in the X-ray beam angle.

Implications

Transient crown discolouration (red or grey) may occur.

The apical portion of the fractured root commonly maintains its neurovascular supply and vitality.

Periodontal pocketing to the fracture line (Figure 11.7) or extrusion of the coronal portion are indicators of poor prognosis.

Management options

1 For coronal fragments that have been completely avulsed, please see Chapter 10 for options on restoring the apical root portion.
2 For apical and middle third root fracture:
a. Administer local anaesthesia.
b. Rinse the area and root surface with saline.
c. Reposition the coronal tooth fragment.
d. Take a radiograph to check the tooth is correctly repositioned.
e. Apply a passive flexible splint to the injured tooth (teeth) as described in Chapter 20 for four weeks (Figure 11.8).
f. Provide post-operative instructions as advised in Chapter 21.
3 For cervical third root fractures, steps 1 to 4 should be followed then:
a. Splint for up to four months (Figure 11.9).
b. Provide post-operative instructions as advised in Chapter 21.

Follow-up

Clinical pulp testing and radiographic examination are recommended at 4, 6-8, 16, 24 weeks, 1 year, and annually thereafter for 5 years.

Prognosis at one year

Negative indicators for the pulp status include mature root formation, displacement, mobility, the distance between the fractured portions, and periapical pathology.

Pulp necrosis of the coronal portion occurs in approximately 20–40% of cases and, therefore will require endodontic intervention but only to the fracture line.

Pulp canal sclerosis occurs in approximately 25% of cases, and therefore discolouration may occur.

Loss of the coronal fragment is more likely with a cervical third fracture (Andreasen et al. 2004, 2012).

KEY POINTS

- Apical and middle third fractures are splinted for 4 weeks.
- Cervical third fracture are splinted for up to 4 months.
- Follow up at 4, 6-8, 16, and 24 weeks, 1 year, and annually thereafter for 5 years.
- Only if the coronal pulp loses vitality should endodontic treatment be initiated; obturation should stop at the fracture line.
- If there is periodontal pocketing or a gingival fenestration, the tooth has a hopeless prognosis.

12 Alveolar process fracture

Figure 12.1 Illustration of an alveolar process fracture, note the fracture is continuous with the labial and palatal cortical plate.

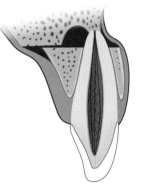

Figure 12.2 Clinical appearance of (a) an alveolar process fracture of the mandibular incisors, (b) the same injury from an occlusal view. (c) Maxillary right central, lateral and left central incisors with an alveolar process fracture. Note the soft tissue tears.

(a)

(c)

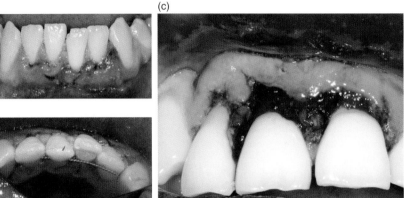

(b)

Figure 12.3 (a) periapical radiograph illustrating the faint outline of the alveolar process fracture (b) occlusal radiograph illustrating the fracture more clearly.

(a)   (b)

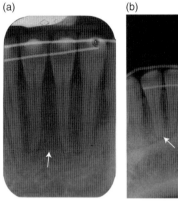

Figure 12.4 Cone beam CT images of an alveolar process fracture in (a) axial section section showing the step in the labial alveolus and (b) sagittal section showing the alveolar fracture is continuous from the labial to the lingual.

(a)   (b)

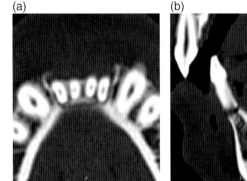

Figure 12.5 (a) Clinical appearance of the mandibular incisors repositioned using digit pressure and subsequent splinting. (b) the occlusion is not affected by the injury nor the splint position.

(a)

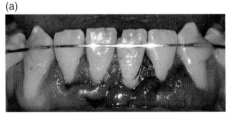

(b)

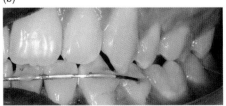

(c) Clinical appearance of the dental hard and soft tissues after 4 weeks of splinting the mandibular incisors.

(c)

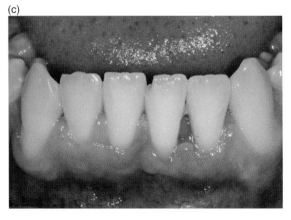

Definition
This injury is a complete fracture of the alveolar process from labial to palatal/lingual cortex, which may or may not involve the alveolar socket (Figure 12.1).

Aetiology
Alveolar fractures usually occur from a significant impact, such as interpersonal violence or a road traffic accident. It accounts for only 3% of all dental injuries. The maxilla is most commonly affected and frequently associated with soft tissue injuries (Andreasen and Lauridsen 2015; Lauridsen et al. 2016).

Clinical examination
- The patient usually presents with significant discomfort in the injured area.
- Visual inspection usually reveals a displaced segment of adjacent teeth with an associated soft tissue tear (Figure 12.2).
- Palpation of the surrounding gingiva usually reveals a step in the bony contour indicating the fracture line.
- Testing mobility of one of the displaced teeth results in the entire segment of displaced teeth moving in unison. This is the classic sign of an alveolar fracture.
- Percussion of the teeth in the fractured segment results in a dull sound in comparison to the adjacent non-traumatised teeth.
- Occlusal disturbance is common; the patient is unable to bite together normally because of the displaced segment.

Pulp test findings
These can be inconclusive for up to three months.

Pulp testing should be repeated during follow-up and only if a persistent negative response is recorded should pulp necrosis be considered in combination with the full clinical picture.

Radiographic findings
Periapical and occlusal radiographs are recommended to visualise the fracture line (Figure 12.3)

A horizontal fracture line can occur at any level of the root length.

To differentiate between a root fracture and alveolar fracture, the alveolar fracture line will move up or down the root length according to the change in the X-ray beam angle. A root fracture will not change in position with a change in the X-ray beam angle.

An additional panoramic tomogram can help visualise the course of the fracture. In some instances, cone beam CT imaging may be of further benefit (Figure 12.4).

Implications
The bony fracture and any associated luxation can compromise the blood supply to the affected teeth and damage the periodontal ligament.

If the displacement is significant, the segment may need to be surgically repositioned.

Management options
a. Administer local anaesthesia.
b. With digit pressure, dis-impact the root apices by moving the teeth in a coronal direction first.
c. Again, with digit pressure supporting the labial and lingual surfaces with your index finger and thumb, respectively, reposition the teeth in alignment with the adjacent teeth.
d. The apices of the injured teeth should return to their sockets. This can be felt by palpating over the area with your thumb as you reposition the teeth. Further instruction on repositioning teeth can be found in Chapter 18.
e. Check the occlusion.
f. Apply a flexible splint to the injured segment and recheck the occlusion described in Chapter 20 for four weeks (Figure 12.5).
g. Suture any soft tissue lacerations.
h. Provide post-operative instructions advised in Chapter 21.

Complications
If the mobile segment of teeth does not reposition with firm digit pressure, assistance from an oral or maxillofacial surgery colleague needs to be sought for an open reduction of the fracture.

Follow-up
Clinical pulp testing and radiographic examination (Figure 12.5) is recommended at 4, 6-8, 16, and 24 weeks, 1 year, and annually thereafter for 5 years.

Prognosis at one year
Pulp necrosis occurs in approximately 35% of cases, and therefore, will require endodontic intervention.

Pulp canal sclerosis occurs in approximately 7% of cases, and therefore discolouration may occur.

Root resorption is rare unless a concomitant luxation injury is present (Andreasen et al. 2011).

KEY POINTS
- A mobile segment of two or more adjacent teeth is a key indicator of an alveolar fracture.
- If the segment does not reposition, an open reduction needs to be considered.
- Splint the repositioned segment for four weeks.
- Follow up at 4, 6-8, 16, and 24 weeks, 1 year, and yearly thereafter for 5 years.

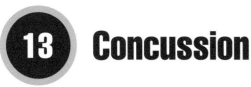

13 Concussion

Figure 13.1 Illustration of a concussion injury.

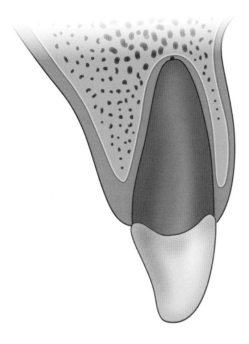

Figure 13.2 (a) Clinical appearance of a concussion injury of the maxillary right central incisor from the facial aspect and (b) the occlusal aspect.

(a)

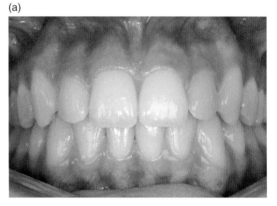

(b)

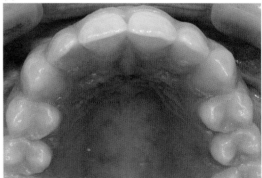

Figure 13.3 Occlusal radiographic appearance of a concussion injury of the maxillary right central incisor. Note the normal appearance of the crown, root, periodontal ligament and periapical tissue.

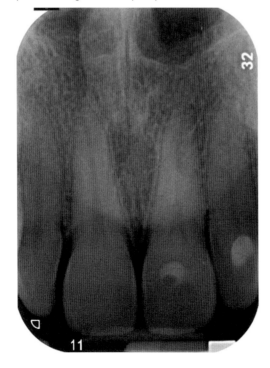

Definition

A concussion injury is confined to the supporting structures of the tooth only (Figure 13.1).

Aetiology

Concussion injuries occur as a result of a direct impact. They occur in approximately 23% of dental injuries (Borum and Andreasen 2001).

Clinical examination

- The patient may present with discomfort to pressure.
- Visual inspection will not identify the injury. Likewise, there will be no displacement of the tooth (Figure 13.2).
- Palpation will not detect any steps in the alveolus or tenderness.
- Mobility will not be present.
- Percussion of the tooth will be uncomfortable for the patient.
- Occlusion will not be altered.

Pulp test findings

Should provide a positive response.

Pulp testing should be repeated during follow-up as an initial negative response indicates an increased risk of pulp necrosis in the future. Only if a persistent negative response is recorded should pulp necrosis be considered in combination with the full clinical picture.

Radiographic findings

Periapical and occlusal radiographs are recommended.

There will be no radiographic abnormalities. The tooth and socket anatomy will be intact (Figure 13.3).

Implications

The impact results in injury and oedema within the periodontal ligament, which results in tenderness to percussion.

Management

a. No treatment is needed.
b. Post-operative instructions as advised in Chapter 21.

Follow-up

Clinical pulp testing and radiographic examination are recommended at 4 weeks and 1 year.

Prognosis at one year

Pulp complications are rare.

Root resorption is very rare and related to repair.

If initial pulp tests are negative, the incidence of pulp necrosis and pulp canal obliteration increases.

If associated with concomitant injuries such as a crown fracture, the risk of pulp and periodontal complications will increase (Hermann et al. 2012; Lauridsen et al. 2012).

KEY POINTS

- Concussion is an injury to the periodontal ligament.
- The tooth will be tender to percussion.
- This alone is not an indication of endodontic intervention.
- Follow up at 4 weeks and 1 year.

14 Subluxation

Figure 14.1 Illustration of a subluxation injury.

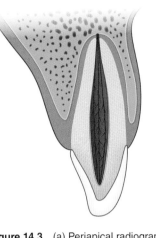

Figure 14.2 Clinical appearance of a subluxation injury to the lower left lateral incisor. Note the bleeding from the gingival sulcus.

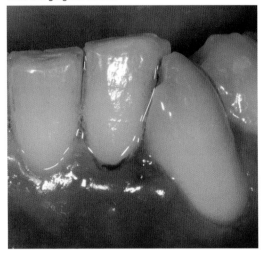

Figure 14.3 (a) Periapical radiograph of a subluxation injury to the mandibular left lateral incisor. (b) Occlusal radiograph of the same mandibular left lateral incisor. Note the normal appearance of the crown, root, periodontal ligament and periapical tissue.

(a)   (b)

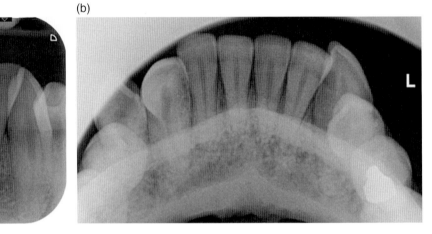

Figure 14.4 Occlusal radiograph of a subluxation injury to the left maxillary central incisor. Note the incidental finding of a middle third root fracture on the adjacent right central incisor, a key reason to take the supplemental occlusal radiograph.

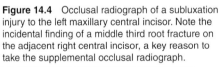

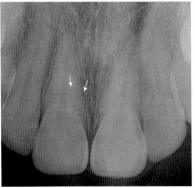

Definition
A subluxation injury causes damage to the tooth's supporting structures, resulting in increased mobility without displacement. Bleeding from the gingival sulcus confirms the diagnosis (Figure 14.1).

Aetiology
Subluxation injuries are a result of a direct impact. They occur in approximately 21% of dental injuries (Borum and Andreasen 2001).

Clinical examination
- The patient may present with discomfort to pressure.
- Visual inspection will detect bleeding from the gingival sulcus. This is the confirmatory factor, indicating damage to the periodontal ligament with tearing of the fibres (Figure 14.2).
- Palpation will not detect any steps in the alveolus or tenderness.
- Mobility in the horizontal direction of the injured tooth will be increased.
- Percussion of the tooth will be uncomfortable for the patient.
- There will be no displacement of the tooth.
- Occlusion will not be altered.

Pulp test findings
It should provide a positive response.

Pulp testing should be repeated during follow-up as an initial negative response indicates an increased risk of pulp necrosis in the future. Only if a persistent negative response is recorded should pulp necrosis be considered in combination with the full clinical picture.

Radiographic findings
Periapical and occlusal radiographs are recommended.

There will be no radiographic abnormalities. The tooth and socket anatomy will be intact (Figure 14.3).

However, the occlusal radiograph may indicate additional asymptomatic injuries; note the incidental middle third root

fracture on the adjacent maxillary right central incisor (Figure 14.4).

Implications
The impact results in haemorrhage and oedema within the periodontal ligament. In rare cases, this may result in rupture of the pulp neurovascular supply.

Management
a. No treatment is needed.
b. For patient comfort, you may consider a flexible splint for 2 weeks.
c. Post-operative instructions as advised in Chapter 21.

Follow-up
Clinical pulp testing and radiographic examination are recommended at 2, 12, 24 weeks, and 1 year.

Prognosis at one year
Pulp necrosis is rare in approximately 12% of cases.

Root resorption is very rare; approximately 3% of cases and related to the repair.

If initial pulp tests are negative, the incidence of pulp necrosis and pulp canal obliteration increases.

If associated with concomitant injuries such as a crown fracture, the risk of pulp and periodontal complications increase as does the incidence of pulp canal obliteration (Hermann et al. 2012; Lauridsen et al. 2012).

KEY POINTS
- Subluxation is an injury to the periodontal ligament.
- Bleeding from the gingival sulcus confirms the diagnosis.
- The tooth will be tender to percussion and mobile.
- This alone is not an indication for endodontic intervention.
- Follow up at 2, 12, and 24 weeks and 1 year.

15 Extrusive luxation

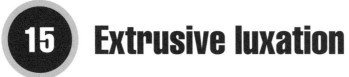

Figure 15.1 Illustration of an extrusion injury.

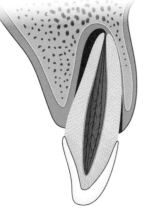

Figure 15.2 Clinical appearance of an extrusion injury of the maxillary right central incisor with associated soft tissue injury to the midline papillae (a) note the crown palatally positioned as well as the incised edge discrepancy. (b) Palatal view demonstrating the periodontal pocketing. (c) lateral view showing the disclusion of the molar teeth due to the premature contact with the central incisor.

(a)

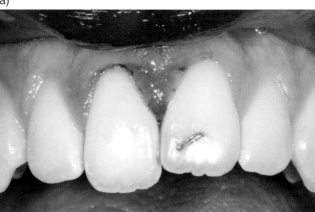

Figure 15.3 Occlusal radiograph of the maxillary anterior teeth illustrating the displaced apex of the right incisor. The radiolucency is not periapical pathology but the alveolar housing of the displaced apex. Note no other adjacent injuries.

(b)

(c)

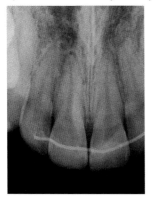

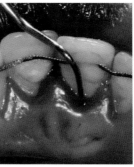

Figure 15.5 Periapical radiograph of the maxillary right central incisor correctly repositioned into its alveolar housing. Note there is now no periapical radiolucency.

Figure 15.4 Clinical appearance of the repositioned maxillary right central incisor. Note the symmetrical incisal edges and the crown is aligned in a bucco-palatal aspect.

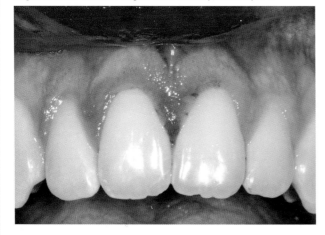

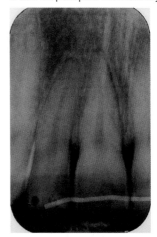

Dental Trauma at a Glance, First Edition. Aws Alani and Gareth Calvert. © 2021 John Wiley & Sons Ltd. Published 2021 by John Wiley & Sons Ltd.
Companion website: www.wiley.com/go/alani/dental_trauma

Definition

An extrusion injury is partial displacement of the tooth out of its socket. The periodontal ligament is partially or totally severed (Figure 15.1).

Aetiology

Extrusion injuries are a result of a direct impact. They occur in approximately 7% of dental injuries (Borum and Andreasen 2001).

Clinical examination

- Visual inspection will confirm the injured tooth appears elongated with an incisal edge position discrepancy, and the crown palatally positioned (Figure 15.2).
- Palpation may detect a hard tissue depression above the apex.
- Mobility in the horizontal and vertical direction of the injured tooth will be obvious.
- Percussion of the tooth may be uncomfortable for the patient.
- Bleeding from the gingival sulcus is due to periodontal ligament damage (Figure 15.2).
- Periodontal pocketing may be present (Figure 15.2).
- Occlusion will be affected as the patient is unlikely to be able to bite normally. (Figure 15.2)

Pulp test findings

Minor extrusion injuries may respond positively.

However, the majority will likely be non-responsive initially.

Therefore, pulp testing should be repeated during follow-up as an initial negative response may indicate an increased risk of pulp necrosis and healing complications in the future. Only if a persistent negative response is recorded should pulp necrosis be considered in combination with the full clinical picture.

Radiographic findings

Periapical and occlusal radiographs are recommended.

There will be a significant widening of the periodontal ligament apically (Figure 15.3).

The alveolar socket will be intact.

Implications

As well as the damage to the periodontal ligament, the neuro-vascular supply to the pulp is severed.

Management

a. You may wish to consider local anaesthesia though it is not always necessary.
b. Clean the exposed root surface with saline.
c. Using a thumb and forefinger support the tooth.
d. Apply pressure in an apical direction, reposition the tooth back into its socket (Figure 15.4).
e. Check the incisal edge and bucco-palatal position.
f. Check the occlusion.
g. Take a periapical radiograph to confirm the tooth has been repositioned (Figure 15.5).
h. Apply a flexible splint for 2 weeks, as described in Chapter 20.
i. Provide post-operative instructions advised Chapter 21.

Follow-up

Clinical pulp testing and radiographic examination are recommended at 2, 4, 8, 12, and 24 weeks, 1 year, and yearly thereafter for 5 years.

Future management

Pulp testing may be inconclusive for up to three months.

If there are at least two signs of pulp necrosis, endodontic treatment should be instigated appropriate to the tooth's stage of root development.

Prognosis at one year

Pulp necrosis occurs in approximately 55% of cases.

If the pulp does revascularise, pulp canal obliteration occurs in approximately 21% of cases.

Surface root resorption occurs in approximately 27% of cases.

Bone loss occurs in approximately 17% of cases.

If associated with concomitant injuries such as a crown fracture, the risk of pulp necrosis increases significantly (Hermann et al. 2012; Lauridsen et al. 2012).

KEY POINTS

- Extrusion injuries make the injured tooth appear elongated.
- The injured tooth is mobile in both an axial and horizontal direction.
- Reposition and place a flexible splint for 2 weeks.
- Follow up at 2, 4, 8, 12, and 24 weeks, 1 year, and yearly thereafter for 5 years.

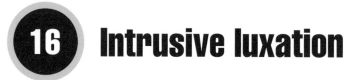

16 Intrusive luxation

Figure 16.1 Illustration of an intrusion injury.

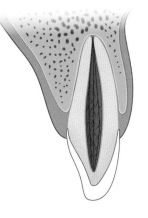

Figure 16.2 (a) Clinical appearance of a severe intrusion injury of the maxillary right central incisor, note the associated soft tissue damage. (b) Clinical appearance of a severe intrusion injury of the left lateral incisor, note the soft tissue dehiscence with exposure of the fractured buccal alveolar plate.

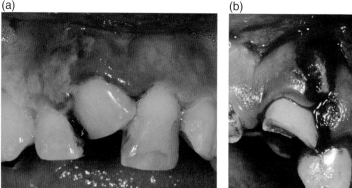

(a)   (b)

Figure 16.3 (a) Periapical and (b) occlusal radiographic appearance of the maxillary right central incisor intrusion injury. Note the apical position of the cemento-enamel junction compared to the adjacent teeth and the periodontal ligament is not visible.

(a)   (b)

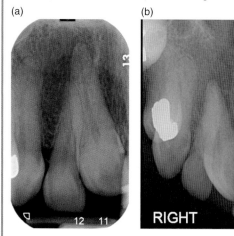

RIGHT

Figure 16.4 Clinical appearance of forceps being used to reposition the intruded maxillary right central incisor. Intrusion injuries tend to be unstable and slip back into their intruded position during manipulation. Note the addition of composite to the incisal edge for better purchase of the incisor preventing damage of the CEJ with the forceps.

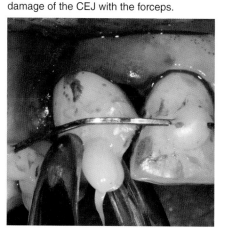

Figure 16.5 Clinical appearance of the the maxillary right central incisor splinted in position.

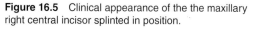

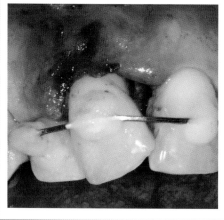

Figure 16.6 Clinical appearance of the intruded maxillary right central incisor at review. Note the soft tissue recession.

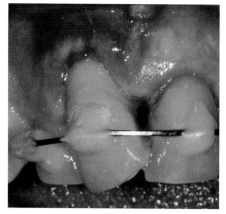

Dental Trauma at a Glance, First Edition. Aws Alani and Gareth Calvert. © 2021 John Wiley & Sons Ltd. Published 2021 by John Wiley & Sons Ltd.
Companion website: www.wiley.com/go/alani/dental_trauma

Definition

An intrusion injury is the displacement of the tooth apically into the alveolar bone. It is associated with a fracture of the alveolar socket (Figure 16.1).

Aetiology

Intrusion injuries are usually a result of falls and cycling accidents. They are rare and occur in approximately 2% of dental injuries (Andreasen et al. 2006b).

Clinical examination

- Visual inspection will confirm the injured tooth is shortened in length due to its more apical position and incisal edge position discrepancy (Figure 16.2a).
- Palpation will detect a hard tissue bulbosity of the alveolar ridge.
- Mobility will not be present; the tooth will be immobile.
- Percussion of the tooth may make a high pitched tone similar to ankolytic changes (replacement resorption) and be uncomfortable for the patient.
- Bleeding from the gingival sulcus may be present or gingival dehiscence with exposure of the alveolar buccal plate (Figure 16.2b).
- Occlusion will not be affected.

Pulp test findings

The injured tooth will likely not respond.

Pulp testing can be repeated during follow-up, but pulp necrosis is very likely to occur for those teeth with complete root formation.

Radiographic findings

Periapical and occlusal radiographs are recommended.

The cementoenamel junction will be more apically positioned than the adjacent non injured teeth, or in some instances, apical to the marginal bone level.

The periodontal ligament will be partially or totally obliterated (Figure 16.3).

Implications

This is a complex injury resulting in damage to all components of the dentoalveolar complex. The severe crushing of the periodontal ligament, neurovascular bundle, and alveolar housing will compromise healing and elicit healing complications.

Emergency management options

1 For intrusion of up to 3 mm
  a. Allow spontaneous re-eruption as this minimises healing complications.
  b. Monitor for 8 weeks.
  c. If no re-eruption occurs, initiate orthodontic or surgical repositioning and apply a flexible splint for 4 weeks.
2 For more severe intrusion
  a. Administer local anaesthesia.
  b. Clean the area with water, saline, or chlorhexidine.
  c. Attempt to grasp the crown with gauze and digital pressure. If unsuccessful, consider grasping the crown wrapped in gauze with forceps and see if the movement can be achieved.
  d. If this is challenging, use gauze or temporarily place flowable composite to the crown for purchase (Figure 16.4).
  e. Avoid grasping the tooth at the cementoenamel junction, as this may provoke healing complications.
  f. Dis-impact the apex by moving the tooth coronally; this will happen suddenly.
  g. The injured tooth will be significantly mobile.
  h. Reposition the tooth to the appropriate apico-coronal level.
  i. Check the patient can occlude as normal.
3 For intrusion such that the crown is not visible
  a. If the crown of the injured tooth is not visible, consider a surgical approach to expose the crown. This may require an onward referral.
  b. Proceed to reposition with forceps, as previously described.
4 Splinting
  a. Apply a flexible splint (Figure 16.5) for 4 weeks as described in Chapter 20.
  b. Suture any gingival laceration.
  c. Take a periapical radiograph to confirm the tooth has been repositioned.
  d. Provide post-operative instructions as advised in Chapter 21.
5 For delayed presentation of minor intrusion injuries
  a. Consider orthodontic extrusion. This can help repair of marginal bone.

Follow-up

Clinical and radiographic examination is recommended at 2, 4, 8, 12, 24 weeks, 1 year, and yearly thereafter for 5 years.

Future management

Teeth with complete root formation will require endodontic intervention within 2 weeks.

A short period of intracanal dressing is advised to reduce the chances of unwanted infection-related resorption. Single-visit endodontics may be less favourable.

Prognosis at one year

Pulp necrosis occurs in all intrusion cases with mature root formation; thus, endodontic treatment is indicated.

Replacement resorption occurs in approximately 10% of cases.

Inflammatory resorption occurs in approximately 5% of cases.

Hard and soft tissue loss occurs in approximately 52% of cases (Figure 16.6).

Over the longer term, the incidence of these complications all increase. As such one in three teeth are lost at 10 years (Andreasen et al. 2006; Wigen et al. 2008).

KEY POINTS

- Mild intrusion less than 3 mm can be allowed to re-erupt.
- Acute management of significant intrusion requires repositioning and a flexible splint for 4 weeks.
- Intruded teeth with mature root formation require endodontic treatment started within 2 weeks. An intracanal medicament is advised for a short period.
- Follow up at 2, 4, 8, 12, 24 weeks, 1 year, and yearly thereafter for 5 years.

17 Lateral luxation

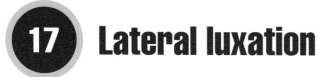

Figure 17.1 Illustration of a lateral luxation injury.

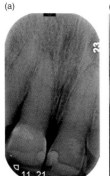

Figure 17.2 Clinical appearance of the laterally luxated maxillary left central incisor from the (a) frontal aspect and (b) the occlusal aspect. Note how there is a bulbosity of the labial buccal plate indicating the displaced root and alveolar fracture. In this case there is an associated gingival tear.

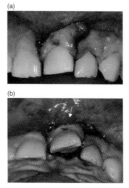

Figure 17.3 Clinical appearance of the maxillary central incisors palatally luxated from the (a) occlusal aspect (b) note there is no posterior occlusal contact.

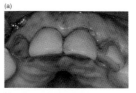
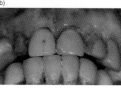

Figure 17.4 (a) Periapical radiograph of the palatally luxated maxillary central incisors (b) Occlusal radiograph of the same maxillary central incisors. Note this view shows the root apex displacement much better (c) as seen in the cone beam CT axial slice.

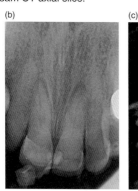

Figure 17.5 Clinical appearance of how to reposition luxated teeth. Grasp the tooth in gauze with your thumb and forefinger, if forceps are required do not hold the CEJ. Support the root apex labially with the finger of your other hand. Apply pressure in a coronal direction only, this dislodges the impacted apex. The tooth mobility will increase. Then bodily reposition the tooth into the correct alignment.

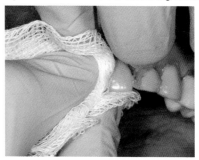

Figure 17.6 Clinical appearance of the now repositioned maxillary central incisors from the (a) occlusal aspect (b) note how the posterior occlusion is now re-established.

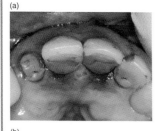
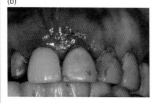

Figure 17.7 Clinical appearance of the now repositioned laterally luxated maxillary left central incisor from the (a) frontal aspect and (b) the occlusal aspect. Clinical appearance of the (c) splinted laterally luxated maxillary left central incisor and sutured soft tissue wound. (d) Review of the injury, note the soft tissue scarring that could be confused as a sinus.

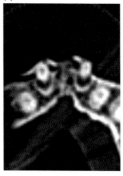

Dental Trauma at a Glance, First Edition. Aws Alani and Gareth Calvert. © 2021 John Wiley & Sons Ltd. Published 2021 by John Wiley & Sons Ltd.
Companion website: www.wiley.com/go/alani/dental_trauma

Definition

A lateral luxation injury is the displacement of the tooth in a labial or palatal direction. It is associated with a fracture of either the labial or palatal alveolar plate (Figure 17.1).

Aetiology

Lateral luxation injuries can be caused by various accidents or interpersonal violence. They are rare and occur in approximately 11% of dental injuries (Borum and Andreasen 2001).

Clinical examination

- Visual inspection will confirm the injured tooth is displaced from its socket laterally (Figure 17.2) or palatally (Figure 17.3).
- Palpation of the root apex will reveal its displacement and a bulge in the labial contour of the alveolus (Figure 17.2).
- Mobility will not be present; the tooth will in fact be immobile.
- Percussion of the tooth will make a high-pitched tone similar to ankylotic changes (replacement resorption) and be uncomfortable for the patient.
- Bleeding from the gingival sulcus or a gingival tear may be present (Figure 17.2).
- Occlusion will likely be affected such the patient cannot close together comfortably on their back teeth (Figure 17.3).

Pulp test findings

The injured tooth is unlikely to respond (Bastos et al. 2014).
   Pulp testing should be repeated during follow-up.

Radiographic findings

Periapical and occlusal radiographs are recommended.
   The injured tooth will appear displaced. The incisal edge will not be level with the adjacent teeth.
   There will be a radiolucency at the root apex. This shows the root apex has been displaced from the alveolar housing. This does not indicate periradicular periodontitis (Figure 17.4).
   A cone beam CT will show how the displaced root apex and fractured labial alveolar plate (Figure 17.4).

Implications

This is a complex injury to the periodontal ligament and alveolus.
   The apex is locked in position between the fractured alveolar plate lateral to the alveolar housing.
   Therefore to reposition the injured tooth, it first must be extruded to disengage the apex from its locked position.

Management

a. Administer local anaesthesia.
b. Clean the area with water, saline, or chlorhexidine.
c. Grasp the crown of the injured tooth with gauze between your thumb and forefinger (Figure 17.5).
d. Support the apex of the injured tooth with a thumb or finger of the other hand, consider instructing your nurse to retract the lips to aide visualisation.
e. Apply pressure in a coronal direction to extrude the tooth, so the apex is no longer locked in place (see Chapter 18).
f. If this movement is not achieved with digit pressure, grasp the injured tooth's crown with gauze and forceps. Do not grasp the crown at the cementoenamel junction.
g. The tooth will then become mobile.
h. Grasping the crown of the tooth with gauze, apply pressure to the crown and simultaneously to the apex to move the tooth back into its original position and alignment (see Chapter 18).
i. Apply pressure to the fractured alveolar plate.
j. Check the patient can occlude as normal (Figure 17.6).
k. Apply a flexible splint for four weeks as described in Chapter 20 (Figure 17.7).
l. Suture any gingival laceration (Figure 17.7).
m. Take a periapical radiograph to confirm the tooth has been repositioned.
n. Provide post-operative instructions as advised in Chapter 21.

For delayed presentation of lateral luxation injuries

1 Follow these same steps, though more pressure may be required to reposition the injured tooth.
2 With significantly delayed presentation, consider orthodontic alignment.

Follow-up

Clinical and radiographic examination is recommended at 2, 4, 8, 12, 24 weeks, one year, and yearly thereafter for five years (Figure 17.7).
   If, there is a continued lack of response from pulp testing, endodontic therapy should be initiated.

Prognosis at one year

Pulp necrosis occurs in approximately 65% of cases.
   Pulp canal obliteration occurs in approximately 13% of cases.
   Surface resorption occurs in approximately 31% of cases.
   Bone loss occurs in approximately 6% of cases.
   Tooth loss is rare.
   If there are adjunctive crown fractures of the luxated tooth, the incidence of these complications increase (Lauridsen et al. 2012a part 1, 2, and 3)

KEY POINTS

- Teeth with lateral luxation injuries have their apex locked in position by the fractured alveolar plate.
- An initial periapical radiolucency demonstrates that the apex has been displaced from the alveolar housing; this is not periradicular periodontitis.
- To reposition the injured tooth, it first needs to be extruded to unlock the apex.
- Splint for 4 weeks.
- Follow up at 2, 4, 8, 12, and 24 weeks, one year, and yearly thereafter for five years.

18 Features of luxation injuries and principles of repositioning

Figure 18.1 Illustration of a luxation injury. Note the displaced root apex lodged between the labial alveolar plate fracture and the original socket.

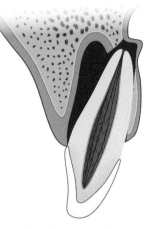

Figure 18.2 (a) Periapical and (b) occlusal radiograph showing a luxated maxillary left central incisor, note the apical displacement is much more obvious in the occlusal view. (c) Cone beam CT radiographic illustration of a luxation injury demonstrating the position of the root apex with respect to buccal alveolar plate and original socket.

(a)

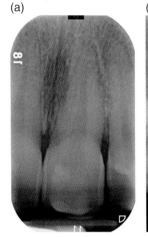

(b)

(c)

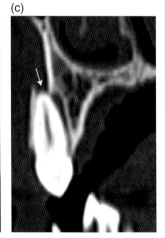

Figure 18.3 Illustration of how to disimpact the apex of a luxated tooth by extrusion.

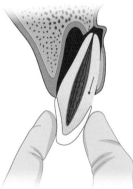

Figure 18.4 Illustration of the dis-impacted apex.

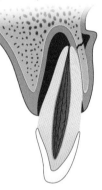

Figure 18.5 Illustration of repositioning the luxated tooth.

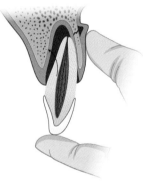

Figure 18.7 (a) Historical palatal luxation injury to the maxillary central incisors having not been repositioned but splinted in their injured position, note the lack of posterior contact due to the early contact on the displaced central incisors (b) the splint was removed, the maxillary central incisors were repositioned with some difficulty and splinted into the correct position, note the re-establishment of posterior contacts.

(a)

(b)

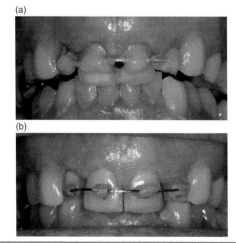

Figure 18.6 Historical luxation injury of the maxillary right lateral incisor having not been repositioned and now compromising the mesio-distal space for replacement of the adjacent missing central incisor.

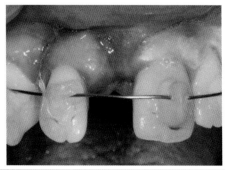

Dental Trauma at a Glance, First Edition. Aws Alani and Gareth Calvert. © 2021 John Wiley & Sons Ltd. Published 2021 by John Wiley & Sons Ltd.
Companion website: www.wiley.com/go/alani/dental_trauma

Features of a luxation injury

Luxation injuries result in the dislodgment of a tooth from its natural position within the arch. This change in position of the tooth, more often than not, results in associated injuries to the alveolar bone and the periodontal ligament (Figure 18.1).

Depending on the magnitude, direction, and vector of the force, hard and soft tissues can either be torn and severed or crushed and compressed. For example, lateral luxation injuries can result in the periodontal ligament being torn on the palatal aspect of the root whilst the buccal alveolar plate is crushed or fractured. It is important for the clinician to appreciate the nature of the injuries as the sequalae of the injuries is likely to reveal itself over time (Figure 18.2).

Crushing injuries

Periodontal ligament

Lateral displacement and intrusion of a tooth will result in marked periodontal ligament cell destruction due to the pressure and force applied to the root.

Teeth with incomplete root development have the potential to spontaneously re-erupt and, therefore, should be given the opportunity to avoid further injury from the repositioning procedure.

Orthodontic repositioning is likely to result in less trauma, but the clinician and patient need to consider the duration of orthodontic treatment, which may last many months or years.

Pulp

The pulp of a tooth with complete root development will have its nerve and blood supply destroyed and will likely require root canal treatment during follow up. The prospect of pulpal revascularization and continued root formation is more favourable in teeth that are optimally repositioned and those with incomplete root development.

Separation injuries

Periodontal ligament

Healing of separation injuries is consistent, but the speed with which this is achieved is related to the ability to reposition the tooth closely to its previous position. The closer the wound margins are after repositioning, the quicker the subsequent healing process.

If the root surface has been contaminated with saliva and not correctly repositioned, there will be a loss of attachment to this portion of the root surface.

Pulp

The ability of the pulp to revascularise is directly related to the success of tooth repositioning, and indeed the apex. For teeth with open apices, the potential for pulp revascularization is greater with optimal repositioning. In immature teeth, a viable Hertwig's epithelial root sheath provides greater potential for continued root and physiological development.

Management

The aim is to:

- Achieve optimal repositioning.
- Promote natural healing of the injuries.
- Restore function and aesthetics.

Suboptimal repositioning is more likely to result in chronic issues for the patient.

Repositioning

a. Administer local anaesthesia.
b. Clean the area with water, saline, or chlorhexidine.
c. Grasp the crown of the injured tooth with gauze in your thumb and forefinger.
d. Apply pressure in a coronal direction to extrude the tooth, so the apex is no longer locked in place (Figure 18.3).
e. If this movement is not achieved with digit pressure, grasp the crown of the injured tooth with gauze and forceps.
f. Do not grasp the cementoenamel junction.
g. The tooth will then become mobile as the apex is no longer locked in place (Figure 18.4).
h. Grasping the crown of the tooth with gauze, apply pressure to the crown and simultaneously to the apex to move the tooth back into its original position and alignment (Figure 18.5).
i. Apply pressure to the fractured alveolar plate.
j. Check the patient can occlude as normal.

Inappropriate or delayed repositioning

When management of a luxation injury is delayed, haemorrhage or an established blood clot within the periodontal ligament and separation injury space make optimal repositioning more challenging.

During the repositioning of injured teeth, there are further micro-traumas taking place. Therefore if the injury is severely delayed and aesthetics/function is not an issue, consideration should be given not to reposition the tooth for risk of further pulp and periodontal damage.

Implications of not repositioning teeth include inadequate prosthetic space for restoration (Figure 18.6) or occlusal disturbance (Figure 18.7).

Sequalae

Where the periodontal ligament and cementum are crushed, the prognosis is much less favourable than those with separation injuries.

Long term sequalae include the development of external cervical root resorption, inflammatory root resorption, replacement resorption, and pulp necrosis.

The development of these conditions may be directly associated with the promptness and efficiency of the initial acute management.

KEY POINTS

- The apex is locked between the fractured alveolar plate and alveolar housing, this stops the tooth from being easily repositioned.
- The prognosis of luxation injuries depends on the severity of the injury and prompt optimal management.
- Separation injuries carry a better prognosis than crushing injuries.

19 Avulsion of a tooth with a closed apex

Figure 19.1 Illustration of an avulsion injury.

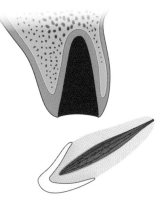

Figure 19.2 Example of a tooth transported in milk.

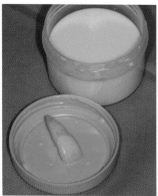

Figure 19.3 Illustration of an avulsed maxillary right central incisor.

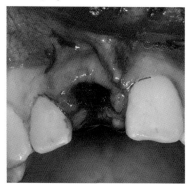

Figure 19.4 Occlusal radiograph demonstrating the small fractures in the buccal plate subsequent to the avulsion of the maxillary central incisors.

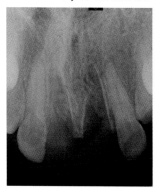

Figure 19.5 Hold the tooth by the crown only.

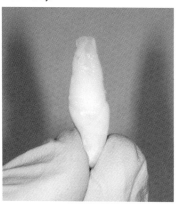

Figure 19.6 Socket irrigation with saline.

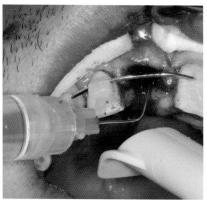

Figure 19.7 (a) Endodontic treatment completed outside the mouth by a second clinician to save time. (b) meanwhile the splint is positioned intra-orally in preparedness once the root canal treatment is completed. (c & d) Avulsed tooth repositioned. (e) Occlusion is confirmed and avulsed tooth is attached to the splint. (f) Periapical radiograph confirming and endodontic. (g) 4 week healing of the avulsed maxillary right incisor.

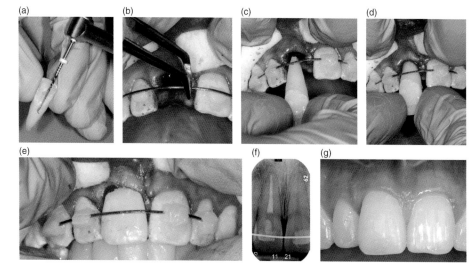

(a)   (b)   (c)   (d)

(e)   (f)   (g)

Dental Trauma at a Glance, First Edition. Aws Alani and Gareth Calvert. © 2021 John Wiley & Sons Ltd. Published 2021 by John Wiley & Sons Ltd.
Companion website: www.wiley.com/go/alani/dental_trauma

Definition

An avulsion injury is when the tooth is completely displaced out of its socket (Figure 19.1).

Aetiology

Avulsion injuries can be caused by various accidents, sporting injuries, and interpersonal violence. Avulsion injuries make up between 0.5–3% of dental injuries (Andersson et al. 2017).

Implications

This is a serious dental injury, and the prognosis is very much dependant on timely management. If the tooth has not been replanted or stored in a suitable storage medium (extraoral dry time) within 60 minutes, the prognosis is extremely poor.

Emergency advice for patients

a. Check if it is a permanent tooth that has been avulsed, primary teeth should not be replanted (Fouad et al. 2020).
b. Find the tooth and pick it up by the crown, not the root.
c. If covered in debris, rinse with milk, saline or the patient's saliva.
d. Replant the tooth gently and bite on a handkerchief.
e. If this is not possible, in descending order of preference store the tooth in a container of milk (Figure 19.2), Hanks balanced storage medium, saliva, saline, or Water (De Brier et al. 2020).
f. Seek emergency dental treatment immediately.

Clinical examination

Visual inspection will confirm the tooth is not in the socket.
  The socket may have debris or coagulum present (Figure 19.3).
  The avulsed tooth will have a mature, closed apex.

Radiographic findings

Periapical and occlusal radiographs are recommended. This will exclude a severe intrusion injury if the tooth is not available
  The socket will be empty.
  There may be evidence of fracture lines in the alveolus (Figure 19.4).

Management options

1 *Tooth replanted prior to arrival at the clinic*
  a. Leave the tooth in place.
  b. Clean the area with saline, water, or chlorhexidine.
  c. Verify the injured tooth is in the correct position clinically and radiographically and there are no other concomitant injuries present.
  d. If the tooth is malpositioned, consider repositioning up to 48 hours after the injury.
  e. Apply a flexible splint (see Chapter 20) for two weeks.
  f. Suture any gingival lacerations.
2 *Tooth extraoral dry time less than 60 minutes*
  Keep the tooth in the storage medium while taking a history and examination
  a. Rinse the root surface with saline while holding only the crown (Figure 19.5).
  b. Administer local anaesthesia – ideally without a vasoconstrictor (Fouad et al. 2020).
  c. Clean the socket and area with saline (Figure 19.6).
  d. If the alveolus is fractured and would impede repositioning of the tooth, this needs correcting with gentle pressure.
  e. Gently reposition the avulsed tooth with digit pressure.

f. Check the occlusion.
g. Verify the injured tooth is in the correct position clinically and radiographically, and there are no other concomitant injuries present.
h. Apply a flexible splint (see Chapter 20) for two weeks.
i. Suture any gingival lacerations.
3 *Tooth extraoral dry time more than 60 minutes*
  The periodontal ligament cells will now be necrotic, but reimplantation is still advised.
  a. Clean the root surface with saline soaked gauze while holding only the crown.
  b. Administer local anaesthesia ideally without a vasoconstrictor.
  c. Clean the socket and area with saline.
  d. If the alveolus is fractured and would impede repositioning of the tooth, this needs correcting with gentle pressure.
  e. Gently reposition the avulsed tooth with digit pressure (Figure 19.7).
  f. Check the occlusion.
  g. Verify the injured tooth is in the correct position clinically and radiographically and there are no other concomitant injuries present.
  h. Apply a flexible splint (see Chapter 20) for two weeks.
  i. Suture any gingival lacerations.

Post-operative care

As well as the post-operative care described in Chapter 21, the following points should be adhered to:
1 Prescribe Amoxicillin. Doxycycline is an alternative but should be avoided in the developing dentition due to the risk of internal staining.
2 Confirm the patient's Tetanus immunisation status.
3 Initiate endodontic therapy within two weeks (Fouad et al. 2020).

Follow up

Endodontic therapy should include a short term inter-visit medicament to try and reduce resorption complications.
  Clinical and radiographic examination is recommended at 2, 4, 12, 24 weeks, one year, and yearly thereafter for five years.
  If replacement resorption occurs, the injured tooth will infra occlude depending on the patient's age; therefore, decoronation may need consideration in the future.

Prognosis at one year with extra alveolar dry time less than 60 minutes

Replacement resorption occurs in approximately 68% of cases.
  Inflammatory root resorption occurs in approximately 21% of cases.
  Bone loss occurs in approximately 7% of cases.
  Tooth loss increases over time, 14% at three years.
  If the extra alveolar dry time is greater than 60 minutes, the incidence of these complications increases (Pohl et al. 2005a, b, c part 1, 2, and 3).

KEY POINTS

- Only hold the crown, do not touch the root.
- The avulsed tooth should be replanted immediately.
- If not, the tooth must be placed in a suitable storage medium like milk.
- In almost all cases the tooth should be replanted irrespective of root development and extraoral dry time.
- Endodontic treatment should be started ideally within two weeks.
- Close observation for infra occlusion and the need for subsequent decoronation is essential.

20 Principles of splinting

Figure 20.1 An example of 0.4mm round stainless steel orthodontic wire for fabrication of a composite wire splint.

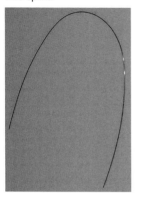

Figure 20.2 An example of a portion of paper clip being used as a composite wire splint in the absence of orthodontic wire.

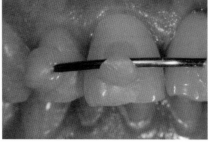

Figure 20.3 An example of a composite fibre splint for the management of trauma to these maxillary incisors. This however is rigid and very difficult to remove.

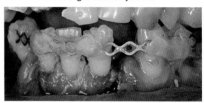

Figure 20.4 An example of a titanium mesh trauma splint. These are very easy to adapt and useful when there are adjacent missing or malaligned teeth in more significant injuries.

Figure 20.5 example of (a) cutting and (b) bending the orthodontic stainless steel wire to (c) the appropriate size and dimension

(a)   (b)   (c)

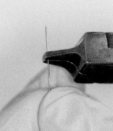
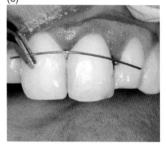

Figure 20.6 (a) application of etch to the traumatised maxillary left central incisor and the teeth either side. (b) Composite added to the adjacent non traumatised incisors. (c) Pre bent stainless steel wire passively set into the composite. (d) Light curing the composite.

(a)   (b)   (c)   (d)

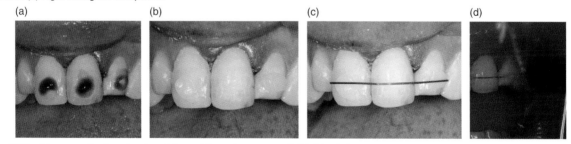

Figure 20.7 (a) composite placed on top of the stainless wire to secure it. (b) Check the position of the traumatised tooth and apply composite to secure the tooth to the wire splint. (c) trimming any excess composite and wire for patient comfort.

(a)   (b)   (c)

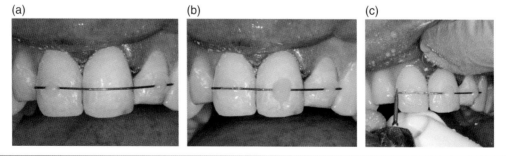

Dental Trauma at a Glance, First Edition. Aws Alani and Gareth Calvert. © 2021 John Wiley & Sons Ltd. Published 2021 by John Wiley & Sons Ltd.
Companion website: www.wiley.com/go/alani/dental_trauma

A splint can be defined as a rigid or flexible device that maintains the position of a displaced or movable part.

For the majority of dental trauma, a passive flexible splint is recommended. This is because rigid fixation of traumatised teeth can result in unfavourable periodontal and pulpal healing (Borssén et al. 2002; Wong and Kolokotsa 2004). It has been suggested that splint mobility allows periodontal remodelling and reduces the potential for replacement resorption (Borssén et al. 2002). Furthermore, prolonged splinting times have shown adverse effects on healing (Borum and Andreasen 2001).

Indications for splinting
- Stabilise traumatised tooth/teeth.
- Increase patient comfort.
- Protection from occlusal forces.
- Facilitate healing.

Contraindications
- Tooth/teeth that are not repositioned.
- Insufficient adjacent non-traumatised teeth.

Ideal properties of a flexible splint
- Easy to construct.
- Passive.
- Flexible in a horizontal and vertical direction.
- Non-irritant to dental soft tissues.
- Easily removable.
- Hygienic and aesthetic.

A composite wire splint fulfils the majority of the factors listed above. Therefore it is the splint of choice. If possible, round orthodontic stainless steel wire 0.016" or 0.4mm should be used (Figure 20.1). On occasion, where the ideal materials cannot be sourced, alternatives may be utilised (Figure 20.2).

Alternatives
- Composite fibre splints (Figure 20.3) can be more aesthetic than a wire-composite splint; however, they are rigid and very difficult to remove and so may result in further complications.

- Titanium trauma splint (Figure 20.4). This is a 0.2mm titanium mesh that is easily manipulated and especially good in situations with adjacent missing or poorly aligned teeth. However, it is significantly more costly than stainless steel.
- Nylon fishing line of 0.13-0.25mm diameter.

Complications of splinting
- Damage of enamel during splint removal – therefore, use of a bonding agent is not recommended.
- Aesthetics – this is a short-term compromise for a long term biological gain.

Step-by-step guide to splinting
a. Reposition the traumatised tooth (teeth) with either digit pressure or forceps, being careful not to grip the CEJ (see Chapter 18).
b. Check the posterior occlusion is correctly established.
c. Take your chosen wire cut roughly to length and bend with pliers or tweezers (Figure 20.5).
d. The splint should include all traumatised teeth in addition to one non-traumatised tooth either side.
e. The splint should be bent such that it is passive when cemented; otherwise, it will apply an orthodontic force to the teeth.
f. Apply etch to the teeth that are to be splinted. Note no bonding agent is necessary as this will make the splint difficult to remove (Figure 20.6).
g. Apply composite to the non-traumatised teeth.
h. Gently and passively set the wire into the composite then light-cure (Figure 20.6).
i. Apply a small amount of composite over the wire to secure it in position and light cure (Figure 20.7).
j. Again, check the injured tooth is in its correct position and have the patient close together to check the occlusion.
k. When happy with the position and occlusion, apply composite to the injured tooth (teeth) to secure to the passive wire splint (Figure 20.7).
l. Trim any excess composite or wire splint (Figure 20.7).

KEY POINTS
- Ensure the posterior occlusion is re-established.
- The splint must be passive when fitted.
- No need to use a bonding agent.
- Consult the most current trauma guidelines for splinting duration.

21 Post-operative instructions

To promote favourable healing and avoid any preventable bacterial biofilm infections, it is important that these post-operative instructions are followed after a dental injury (Bourguignon et al. 2020; Levin et al. 2020).

Pain relief

A liquid form of pain relief, such as dispersible paracetamol, can be more easily consumed in the early stages of healing.

For the first 24 hours, non-steroidal anti-inflammatories such as ibuprofen should be used per the manufacturer's daily dose recommendations. This can start immediately after the emergency treatment and preferably before the local anaesthetic wears off.

If non-steroidal anti-inflammatories are contraindicated, paracetamol, as per the manufacturer's daily dose recommendations, can be taken.

After 24 hours, pain relief medication can be taken when needed.

Swelling

If swelling is present or occurs after 24 hours, a cold compress can be applied for 10 minutes at a time to the area.

Soft diet

For the first 14 days after dental trauma, you should consume a soft diet. This means no hard food but does not necessarily mean a liquidised diet.

Extremes of temperature may be uncomfortable, so avoid anything too hot or too cold.

Oral hygiene

Meticulously clean the teeth, gums, and splint two to three times a day with a small soft toothbrush or single tufted brush.

This should be supplemented with chlorhexidine mouth wash twice a day, especially if some swelling or lacerations prevent mechanical plaque removal with a toothbrush.

Lip balm

For lip lacerations or abrasions, lip balm or petroleum jelly application will prevent dryness.

Antibiotics

A prescription of antibiotics is only indicated for an avulsion injury. This is usually Amoxicillin. Doxycycline is an alternative but should be avoided in the developing dentition due to the risk of internal staining.

Tetanus

If the injury or avulsion has happened in and around soil, a tetanus status update should be sought. This may require a tetanus booster.

Splint loosening

If the splint was to become loose or fall off, an appointment should be made immediately to have the splint repaired.

Prevention

Avoid all contact sports for the recommended healing period relevant to your particular injury.

Follow up

You should attend the dentist at the recommended review intervals, which may include 2, 4, 8, 24, 52 weeks, and yearly thereafter for five years, depending on your injury.

It is essential to detect any healing complications as soon as possible so they can be managed appropriately.

[This page was left blank intentionally]

22 Follow-up and splint removal

Figure 22.1 Clinical appearance of a laceration healing with sutures still in situ that was confused with a sinus.

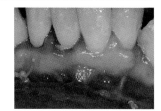

Figure 22.2 Cold test Endo-Frost™ (Coltene) during follow up for the maxillary right central incisor.

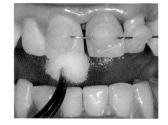

Figure 22.3 Electric pulp tester during follow up for the maxillary left central incisor.

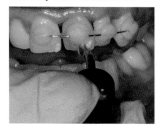

Figure 22.4 Periapical radiograph of the maxillary right central incisor with an area of periapical radiolucency which is not indicative of periradicular disease but a malpositioned apex following a luxation injury.

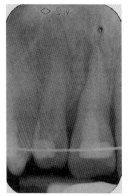

Figure 22.5 Occlusal radiograph showing marginal alveolar breakdown of the maxillary central incisors subsequent to luxation injuries.

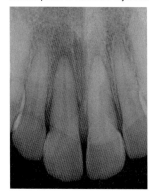

(a)

Figure 22.6 (a) Periapical radiograph showing a mid third horizontal root fracture of the maxillary right canine previously missed and not splinted. (b) More than likely because of the significant and multiple other injuries the patient experienced.

(b)

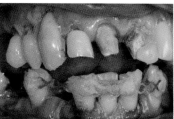

Figure 22.7 (a) Clinical appearance of the mandibular splint at review. (b) High speed diamond bur removing the composite from between the injured central incisor teeth and the wire - leaving the remainder of the splint intact. (c) Now the injured central incisor teeth are independent of the splint they can be tested for mobility and percussion. If there are persistent signs or symptoms the injured central incisors can be easily reattached. (d) Otherwise the remaining composite and wire can be removed.

(a)　　　　(b)

(c)　　　　(d)

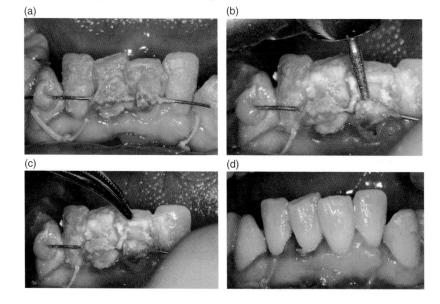

Dental Trauma at a Glance, First Edition. Aws Alani and Gareth Calvert. © 2021 John Wiley & Sons Ltd. Published 2021 by John Wiley & Sons Ltd.
Companion website: www.wiley.com/go/alani/dental_trauma

Follow-up

Regular follow-up is essential to monitor healing such that complications are identified correctly and early.

By identifying complications early, they can be potentially managed in a more conservative manner, having less of an impact on the tooth's need for continued interventions throughout the lifetime of the patient.

The follow-up intervals recommended in this book and elsewhere have a degree of flexibility. An individual rarely experiences just one traumatic injury, there are usually multiple injuries, and therefore the patient's follow-up interval should be based on the most severe injury. A summary of follow-up intervals can be found in Appendix A.

Clinical examination

- Having clinical photographs to monitor soft tissue healing is invaluable as visual inspection may reveal scarring – do not confuse this with swelling or a sinus (Figure 22.1).
- Palpation of the surrounding gingiva may reveal tenderness over an apex or where the alveolar plate was fractured.
- Mobility may or may not be present.
- Percussion of the tooth may be uncomfortable for an extended period of time. This is not a sign of periradicular disease. It is most likely a sign of periodontal ligament damage.

Pulp testing

At each recommended follow-up interval, the traumatised tooth (teeth) and at least one non-traumatised tooth should be tested for comparison.

- Cold test Endo-Frost™ (Coltene), not ethyl chloride (Figure 22.2).
- Electric pulp test (Figure 22.3).

The time delay between administering the test and a positive reaction is not in itself diagnostic of pulpal disease.

What is more important is a consistently negative response in comparison to a non-traumatised tooth or a change in response over the months of review.

One diagnostic test at a one-time point provides a very limited and possibly misleading clinical picture; hence detecting change over a series of follow-up is much more valuable.

Radiographic examination

During the follow-up intervals, periapical or occlusal radiographs are advised for the traumatised and adjacent teeth.

The most common findings early in the follow-up period are:

- A malpositioned apex which can simulate periradicular disease (Figure 22.4).
- Transient apical breakdown which can simulate periradicular disease.
- Marginal bone loss which is self-limiting (Figure 22.5).

Again, having multiple time frames for comparison builds a better diagnostic picture than a single radiographic image.

Unfortunately, injuries can be missed for a variety of reasons and don't become apparent until follow-up (Figure 22.6).

If there is a discrepancy between the clinical presentation and the radiographic findings, three-dimensional imaging should be requested.

Splint removal

Splinting times recommended in this book and elsewhere are not absolute. It has been shown 60% of the periodontal ligament mechanical function returns after two weeks, and splinting duration is unlikely to affect this (Mandel and Viidik 1989).

If there are multiple adjacent injuries, the splinting time should be judged using common sense based on the most complex injury.

Likewise, at the time of splint removal, if there is still mobility or significant discomfort, the splinting time can be increased. A good example of this is a cervical third fracture, which can be splinted for up to four months due to the risk of mobility.

Therefore when the time comes to remove a splint, a certain degree of retrievability is helpful (Figure 22.7).

a. For the traumatised tooth (teeth), use a fine diamond bur to section the composite between the tooth and splint.

b. The traumatised tooth can be tested for mobility and percussion independently from the support provided by the splint.

c. If there is persistent mobility and tenderness, the traumatised tooth can be easily secured back to the wire splint with composite for another two weeks.

d. If the injured tooth responds normally, the remaining splint can be removed with a diamond and then tungsten carbide bur.

Pulp healing

Every effort should be made to preserve the pulp of an immature tooth. Occasionally in crushing injuries, apical pulp healing may present as an apical radiolucency. Given a short period, this will resolve.

The strongest predictors for pulp necrosis are the extent of displacement and size of the apical foramen.

This is followed by compression/crushing of the apical tissue, external contamination, dentine exposure, and pulpal exposure.

Periodontal healing

If the area of damage is small, the periodontal ligament has the capacity to heal. If larger areas are damaged, resorption may occur as described in Chapters 27 and 28.

Factors that affect this are crushing injuries and drying out of the cells from avulsion.

Due to the surface area and sensitivity of the periodontal ligament, tenderness to percussion can be present for many years after dental trauma.

Alveolar healing

Breakdown of the marginal bone can occur following luxation, intrusion, alveolar fractures, and late or unsuccessful repositioning.

This is detected radiographically (Figure 22.5) or, in severe cases, clinically with marked gingival recession.

KEY POINTS

- Regular follow-up is key to the success of treatment and managing complications that may flow from the original trauma.
- Awareness of the physiologic and pathologic processes that are ongoing will help the clinician to decide which signs need active management and treatment.
- Splinting times are a general guide-clinician discretion should be exercised depending on the severity and complexity of the presenting injury.

23 Indications for endodontic treatment

Figure 23.1 (a) Healing soft tissue laceration that was mistaken for a sinus after (b) dental trauma associated with the maxillary left central incisor.

(a)

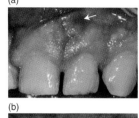

(b)

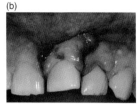

Figure 23.2 (a) A PCP-12 periodontal probe locating an isolated periodontal pocket to the depth of horizontal root fracture associated with the maxillary left central incisor rendering endodontic treatment hopeless. Note the soft tissue swelling and the mucogingival junction. (b) The occlusal radiograph of the same maxillary left central incisor identifying the pathology associated with middle third root fracture.

(a)   (b)

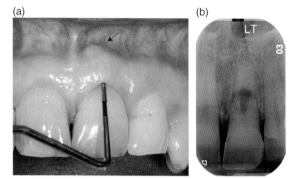

Figure 23.3 (a) Periapical radiograph showing an enamel-dentine crown fracture of the maxillary left incisor with an immature root form and the suggestion of a periapical radiolucency. (b) Given time and regular follow up the root has continued to form with no sign of of periapical pathology - endodontic treatment was never required.

(a)   (b)

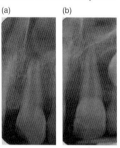

Figure 23.4 (a) Occlusal radiograph showing a middle third root fracture of the maxillary left incisor that has developed pulp necrosis of the coronal portion (b) endodontic treatment completed to the fracture line with a bioceramic obturation material.

(a)   (b)

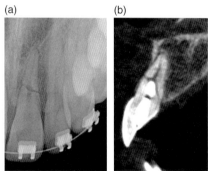

Figure 23.5 (a) Clinical appearance of a maxillary right central incisor with an enamel-dentine-pulp fracture and associated sinus at the mucogingival junction. (b) Periapical radiograph of the same central incisor post endodontic treatment, note the lack of periapical pathology. (c) Occlusal radiograph of the maxillary central incisor identifying the previously missed middle third root fracture and reason for the sinus at the mucogingival junction. (d) Clinical picture of the apical root fragment and obturation removed with endodontic microsurgery. (e) 1 year follow up periapical radiograph of the right central incisor showing complete healing

Figure 23.6 A clinical example of carrying out endodontic treatment of an avulsed central incisor that has been out of the mouth more than 60 minutes. Note the tooth is held by the crown only, this can be challenging.

(a)   (b)   (c)

(d)   (e)

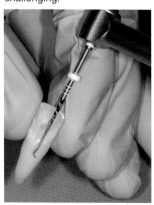

Dental Trauma at a Glance, First Edition. Aws Alani and Gareth Calvert. © 2021 John Wiley & Sons Ltd. Published 2021 by John Wiley & Sons Ltd.
Companion website: www.wiley.com/go/alani/dental_trauma

Definition

Endodontic treatment aims to prevent or resolve pulpal and periradicular disease. A necrotic pulp may occur due to the invasion of bacteria or rupture of the neurovascular supply.

Endodontic diagnosis for traumatised teeth can be challenging. Decision making based on a single consultation provides a very limited diagnostic picture; therefore, the importance of follow up cannot be underestimated to gather longitudinal data for a more reliable diagnosis (Figure 23.1).

Symptoms

A detailed SOCRATES pain history should be completed. If efficiently done, this alone may give a strong indication of the diagnosis.

Clinical examination

- Visual inspection may identify a colour change of the crown. As discussed in Chapter 25, this is a poor indicator of pulp status.
- Palpation of the root apex may precipitate discomfort or identify swelling; this may be a displacement injury but is also commonly associated with periradicular disease.
- A sinus is indicative of periapical pathology. It is good practice to place a gutta percha point in the sinus for radiographic examination.
- Mobility is a poor indicator of pulpal or periapical health. Mobility is more indicative of fracture or displacement injuries.
- Percussion is a test of the periodontal ligament. As almost all injuries involve damage to the periodontal ligament, tenderness to pressure or percussion is common and not necessarily an indicator of pulpal or periapical disease. In fact, traumatised teeth can be tender to percussion for an extended time after the injury. Therefore, endodontic intervention is not indicated with this test alone. Otherwise, the percussion of teeth can identify a change in percussion tone, indicative of replacement resorption.
- An isolated deep periodontal pocket identified with a PCP-12 periodontal probe is the quintessential indication of a root fracture, either vertical or horizontal (Figure 23.2).
- Occlusal examination may identify fremitus. This occurs when a tooth has a premature contact and moves horizontally to accomodate maximum intercuspation. This may be in conjunction with tenderness to percussion and indicative of a previous displacement injury.

Special tests

Injured teeth can respond negatively for up and beyond to three months before a positive response is noted.

Therefore it is more important to note changes in results over multiple time points and in comparison to an otherwise healthy contralateral tooth.

The combination of an electric pulp and cold test is the most reliable indicator of pulp status (Chen and Abbott 2011).

A cold test is best administered with a refrigerated CO_2 spray, not ethyl chloride.

Radiographs

More than one angle of the radiograph is essential. If the diagnosis is unclear, cone beam CT imaging should be considered.

Commonly, early widening of the periodontal ligament or a periapical radiolucency is a sign that the root apex has been displaced/not repositioned into the alveolar housing, not of periradicular disease (Figure 23.3).

Loss of the lamina dura indicates either intrusion or horizontal root fracture at the acute presentation, or external resorption if identified later.

Reaching a diagnosis

It is recommended that a change in at least two signs, symptoms, or special tests over longitudinal follow up should occur before endodontic intervention is initiated.

Special considerations

Inter-visit medicament

There is a low level of evidence for the prolonged use of inter-visit medication to reduce root resorption. The risks of coronal leakage and fracture resistance reduction in the longer-term outweigh the indication for prolonged dressings.

Horizontal root fracture

Only if the coronal portion of the fractured root becomes necrotic is endodontic treatment indicated. The chemomechanical preparation should stop at the fracture line, and obturation at this point is completed with a biocompatible material (Figure 23.4).

It is unusual for the fractured apical root portion to become necrotic. If it does, periradicular surgery or extraction should be considered (Figure 23.5).

Avulsion

If the extra alveolar dry time is more than 60 minutes, endodontic treatment can be completed out of the mouth. The tooth must be held by the crown, and ironically this makes treatment more challenging than after the tooth is reimplanted (Figure 23.6).

Pulp canal obliteration

This is not an indication for endodontic therapy. Furthermore, the iatrogenic risks of a challenging access must be appreciated (see Chapter 24).

Root resorption

Replacement and external cervical resorption are not indications for orthograde endodontics (see Chapters 27 and 28).

KEY POINTS

- Longitudinal follow-up will highlight changes in signs or symptoms, which is essential for reaching a correct diagnosis.
- Comparison should be drawn with unaffected contralateral teeth.
- Tenderness to percussion is not always a sign of periradicular disease and is persistent in traumatised teeth irrespective of endodontic treatment.
- A periapical radiolucency may be a historic displacement of the root tip from the alveolar housing, not a periradicular disease process.
- A change in at least two signs, symptoms or special tests should occur before endodontic intervention is initiated.

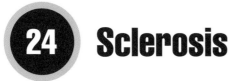

Sclerosis

Figure 24.1 Clinical examples of teeth discoloured by sclerosis (a) maxillary left central incisor extra oral and intra oral views. (b) Maxillary right central incisor extra oral and intra oral views.

(a) (a2)
(b) (b2)

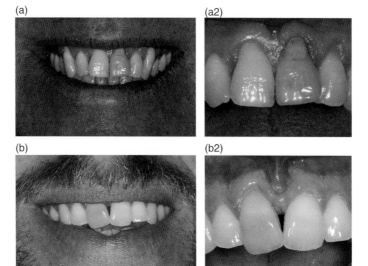

Figure 24.2 Periapical radiograph of a maxillary left central incisor showing sclerosis of the coronal pulp. Note the pulp does become visible apically. Note the normal appearance of the periapical tissue.

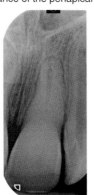

Figure 24.3 Cone beam CT image of sclerosed maxillary right lateral and left central incisors. Note the difference in canal diameters of the incisors. Arrows point toward the patent canal, note it is in the centre of the root form, not off to one side.

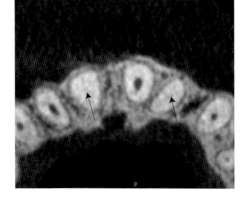

Figure 24.4 Periapical radiograph of a sclerosed maxillary left lateral incisor with excessive tooth tissue loss and perforation during attempted endodontic access. Note the normal appearance of the periapical tissue indicating no periradicular disease.

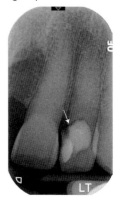

Figure 24.5 Clinical appearance of (a) a sclerosed maxillary right central incisor before single tooth vital bleaching. (b) Post-operative colour change of the bleached vital maxillary right central incisor.

(a) (b)

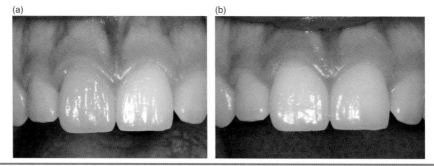

Dental Trauma at a Glance, First Edition. Aws Alani and Gareth Calvert. © 2021 John Wiley & Sons Ltd. Published 2021 by John Wiley & Sons Ltd.
Companion website: www.wiley.com/go/alani/dental_trauma

Definition

Sclerosis or pulp canal obliteration is the deposition of dental hard tissue within the root canal space resulting in a yellow discolouration of the clinical crown (Figure 24.1) (McCabe and Dummer 2012).

Aetiology

Dental trauma can result in pulp canal obliteration, potentially damaging the neurovascular supply of the pulp. The more significant the injury, the more likely pulp canal obliteration is to occur.

The calcification found in the root canal system varies between poorly organised secondary, tertiary dentine, or even osteodentine. There is, however, no inflammatory component.

The discolouration can be apparent from three months after the incident.

Prevalence

Approximately 4–25% of traumatised teeth show signs of pulp canal obliteration. Teeth with luxation injuries or those with immature root development are the most commonly presenting.

The most commonly affected tooth is the maxillary incisor.

Of the teeth with pulp canal obliteration between 7 and 27% (mean of 11%) show signs of periradicular disease after a 21-year follow-up (McCabe 2011). This is more likely if the tooth had a mature apex at the time of injury.

Clinical examination

- Teeth with pulp canal obliteration are generally asymptomatic.
- Visual inspection of the injured tooth will show a more yellowish colour with loss of transparency and darker hue because of the increased volume of tooth mass in the clinical crown.
- There is usually no apical tenderness to palpation.
- There is usually no tenderness to percussion.
- Mobility is within normal physiological limits.

Pulp test findings

As the pulp canal obliteration becomes more pronounced, the distance between the enamel surface and pulp increases; therefore, there will be a progressively reduced response.

This does not indicate pulpal necrosis. A reduced response is still a positive response.

It is important to use a correct cold test; ethyl chloride is not recommended as it does not produce a cold enough temperature.

Radiographic findings

Two periapical radiographs from different angles are recommended.

The root canal system is either partially or completely obliterated with what appears radiographically to be dentine (Figure 24.2).

This does not mean the root canal space is not patent, just that conventional radiography is not sensitive enough to detect it.

There is unlikely to be signs of a periapical radiolucency.

Additional three-dimensional imaging, such as a small field of view using cone beam CT, can be useful if treatment is required (Figure 24.3).

Implications

The increased mass of tooth structure is the reason for the colour change and delayed response to sensitivity testing.

These teeth respond to vital bleaching and do not necessarily require endodontic intervention.

If endodontic treatment is indicated, there is a risk of iatrogenic damage, including excess tooth tissue loss, perforation, and file fracture (Figure 24.4).

Management

Monitor

There is no active management required for the pulp.

Vital bleaching

The affected tooth can be whitened for an extended period that will improve the colour (Figure 24.5).

Restoration

Direct or indirect restorations could be considered, but the aesthetic gain should be balanced by the biological cost of the sacrificed tooth tissue.

Endodontics

Endodontic treatment is only indicated if the patient reports symptoms or there are radiographic signs of periradicular disease as discussed in chapter 23.

Irrespective of the radiographic pulp canal size, there will be a clinically patent lumen.

The root canal system will be located in the middle of the root at the level of the cementoenamel junction.

The access cavity should extend away from the cingulum towards the incisal edge for better visibility and axial access.

The calcified tooth tissue will be a different colour to the axial wall root dentine.

A dental operating microscope with light and magnification will aid root canal location.

Once the canal is accessed, extreme care needs to be exercised not to ledge, block or transport the root canal apically.

Prognosis

Pulp canal obliteration has little effect on tooth retention. Pulp survival is approximately 84% at 20 years

KEY POINTS
- Change in tooth colour is not a reliable indicator of pulpal status.
- Pulp canal obliteration alone is not an indication for endodontic intervention.
- The colour can be improved by vital bleaching.

25 Discolouration

Figure 25.1 Clinical example of sclerosis (pulp canal obliteration) (a) pre operatively and (b) post operatively after vital bleaching of the maxillary left central incisor.

(a)

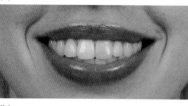

(b)

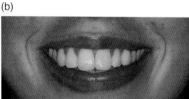

Figure 25.2 Clinical example of a reddish discolouration of the (a) maxillary right lateral incisor very soon after dental trauma, indicating haemorrhage within the pulp space. (b) Periapical radiograph of the maxillary right lateral incisor showing a normal appearance.

(a)   (b)

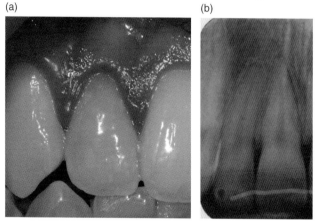

Figure 25.3 Clinical example of pink discolouration from external cervical resorption (a) maxillary right central incisor and (b) maxillary right lateral incisor. (c) Periapical radiograph of the maxillary right central incisor with an invasive cervical resorption lesion.

(a)   (c)

(b)

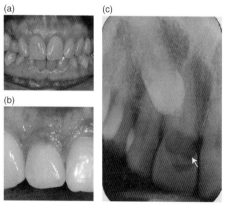

Figure 25.4 Clinical example of (a) the maxillary right canine discoloured from MTA obturation. (b) Improvement in colour following internal-external bleaching. (c) Radiographic appearance of the resorption repair with MTA of the maxillary right canine.

(a)   (c)

(b)

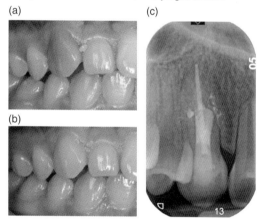

Figure 25.5 (a) Clinical example of a discoloured maxillary left central incisor due to previous root canal treatment. (b) Periapical radiograph of the maxillary left central incisor showing suboptimal obturation.

(a)   (b)

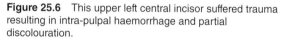

Figure 25.6 This upper left central incisor suffered trauma resulting in intra-pulpal haemorrhage and partial discolouration.

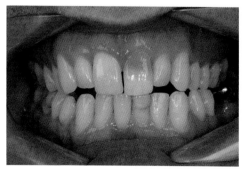

Dental Trauma at a Glance, First Edition. Aws Alani and Gareth Calvert. © 2021 John Wiley & Sons Ltd. Published 2021 by John Wiley & Sons Ltd.
Companion website: www.wiley.com/go/alani/dental_trauma

Definition

Discolouration of teeth is described as any change in the hue, colour, or translucency of the tooth by any cause. Discolouration or staining of a tooth can occur in two ways:

- Intrinsic staining is caused by discolouration from within the tooth structure.
- Extrinsic staining is attached to the external tooth surface.

Aetiology

There are many different causes for the discolouration of teeth, but also many different types of discolouration.

This chapter will focus mainly on the discolouration caused by dental trauma, or its management and long term complications (Krastl et al. 2013).

Intrinsic

Yellow/brown

Up to 25% of teeth with a history of dental trauma show signs of pulp canal obliteration (Figure 25.1). This is because the pulp volume decreases, and the dentine volume increases. This increase in dentine volume affects the optical properties of the tooth, causing yellow dentine discolouration.

As this is not an indicator of pulp necrosis, endodontic treatment is not indicated. The tooth could be monitored, or consideration given to bleaching, direct or indirect veneer (see Chapter 24) (Sulieman 2008).

Red/brown

Dental trauma may lead to the rupture of intrapulpal blood vessels and haemorrhage, which releases blood components into the dentinal tubules causing discolouration (Figure 25.2). The pulp may well recover from this injury, and the discolouration may spontaneously resolve (Malmgren and Hübel 2012).

Treatment options would include radiographic and sensitivity investigations to assess if the pulp is, in fact, necrotic.

Pink

A long term complication of dental trauma is external cervical resorption (Figure 25.3). This can result in a pink spot on the crown of the tooth due to the increasing size of the vascular resorption lesion eroding the tooth's dentine.

Treatment options would include surgical repair or extraction. Occasionally orthograde endodontics is required along with surgical repair.

Grey

Mineral trioxide aggregate (MTA) is a material known for its excellent biocompatibility. Therefore, it is used to pulp-cap complex fractures exposing the pulp or the obturation of wide immature apices. However, a long-term consequence is a grey discolouration in part due to its iron content (Krastl et al. 2013).

Treatment options could include bleaching (Figure 25.4) or a direct/indirect restoration to camouflage the colour (Setien et al. 2008).

Black

Where pulp injury is severe and subsequent root canal treatment is suboptimal, pulp and haemorrhage remnants in combination with biofilm formation due to inadequate chemo-mechanical instrumentation and coronal seal can produce severe black discolouration. (Figure 25.5).

If all other special tests indicate the pulp is necrotic, endodontic treatment (Figure 25.6) with activated sodium hypochlorite irrigation and an optimal coronal seal is recommended. If further improvement in the colour is necessary, internal/external bleaching is a minimally invasive procedure with excellent results.

Extrinsic

Brown

A week of using chlorhexidine mouth wash following dental trauma will cause brown staining to build up on the external enamel surface. This will cease when normal tooth brushing can be comfortably resumed, and the mouthwash is no longer needed.

Treatment of this is extrinsic staining is simple with scaling or air polishing.

Implications

Tooth discolouration is a poor indicator of pulp status and should not be used in isolation as an indicator of endodontic intervention.

KEY POINTS

- Additional special tests should be carried out before concluding a diagnosis of pulp necrosis.
- Discolouration is not always consistent with loss of pulp vitality.
- Bleaching for an extended period is a minimally invasive treatment that can make a significant improvement in appearance without biological sacrifice.

26 Management of the immature root

Figure 26.1 (a) Incidental finding of a maxillary right central incisor with an open apex. (b) Periapical radiograph illustrating the thin root canal walls prone to mechanical failure and the 'blunderbuss' nature of the apex.

(a) (b)

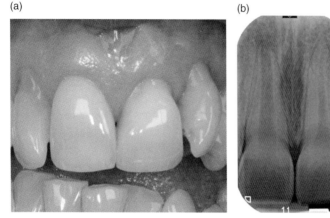

Figure 26.2 Periapical radiograph of a maxillary left lateral incisor with an open apex that had been dressed numerous times with Calcium Hydroxide resulting in extrusion of the dressing into the periradicular tissue.

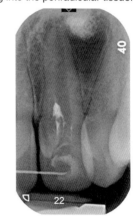

Figure 26.3 Clinical example of a maxillary central incisor with an open apex viewed through the dental operating microscope. The reflective glare at the apex is the moist apical tissue. If the canal cannot be dried a short duration intervisit medicament should be placed and obturation postponed.

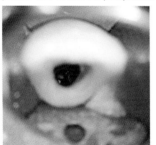

Figure 26.4 Clinical example of a side venting luer lock syringe being measured 2mm short of the confirmed working length to prevent extrusion of sodium hypochlorite.

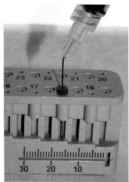

Figure 26.5 Clinical example of a plugger measured to the canal confirmed working length to place mineral trioxide aggregate (MTA).

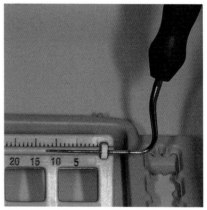

Figure 26.6 Clinical example of the obturation process. (a) MTA being placed into the canal and (b) heated gutta percha placed on top of the 4mm MTA plug under the dental operating microscope.

(a) (b)

Figure 26.7 Periapical radiographs showing (a) pre and (b) post operative MTA placement in immature roots with open apices. Note the resolution of the periapical radiolucencies.

(a1) (a2) (a3)

(b1) (b2) (b3)

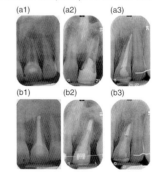

Dental Trauma at a Glance, First Edition. Aws Alani and Gareth Calvert. © 2021 John Wiley & Sons Ltd. Published 2021 by John Wiley & Sons Ltd.
Companion website: www.wiley.com/go/alani/dental_trauma

Acute management

Every effort should be made to retain the pulp vitality of an injured tooth with an immature root form. Therefore they should always be reimplanted where possible, or a pulpotomy as the preferred management of pulp exposure (Chapter 8).

Delayed management

Stunted root formation commonly presents as a result of trauma during the developmental stages of a tooth. The underdevelopment of the root and apex may be further compounded by the presence of a periapical lesion, which may result in resorption of the already compromised structure.

Clinical examination

Teeth commonly present with discolouration due to the long standing necrosis of the pulp and the underdeveloped nature of the root canal system. Other aspects, such as the presence of a draining sinus, are also common. Alternatively, the open apex may be an incidental finding (Figure 26.1).

Radiographic examination

- Thin root canal walls.
- Tapering root canal walls towards a wide apex.
- Well established periapical lesion.
- Historical inter visit medicament extrusion (Figure 26.2).
- Additional cone beam CT imaging may be required to fully visualise the clinical situation three dimensionally.

Establishment of the working length

- Once access is gained to the root canal system, and the majority of necrotic debris is removed, the working length can be established.
- Depending on the size of the apex and its visualisation, the working length can be established by an electronic apex locator.
- Due to the width of the canal, stabilising a file, however large it may be, can be difficult to achieve. The best option is to utilise the largest file that can fit passively and snugly in the canal.
- Alternatively, the use of a large paper point and the identification of moisture or blood at the end of the point can also provide a further avenue for length determination.
- A further option is the use of a large gutta percha point. This will be flexible enough to place within the canal without damaging the walls and maybe more stable when taking a radiograph to establish the length.

Preparation of the open apex

- The preparation method is largely chemical in nature with the aim of either removing micro-organisms physically, through the creation of fluid dynamics or dissolution through the action of the irrigants (Figure 26.3).
- This is largely achieved through irrigation of the canal system with 3–5% sodium hypochlorite.
- The irrigating syringe should be side-venting and measured 2 mm short of the confirmed working length to avoid extrusion injuries (Figure 26.4).
- The irrigant can be placed into the canal and energised with ultrasonic instruments to create sheer stresses at the surface of the root canal to optimise the removal of biofilm.
- Other techniques to optimise irrigation efficiency include the use of a Tepe brush to cleanse the surface of the dentine without frank dentine removal.
- Once sodium hypochlorite irrigation is complete, a rinse with saline and drying can be considered prior to dressing or obturation.

Canal dressing

- Once irrigation and preparation is complete, the clinician needs to consider whether a dressing is required.
- If suppuration or significant moisture is present, a dressing of non-setting calcium hydroxide is advised.
- If there is an absence of moisture within the canal or suppuration, the clinician can instigate root canal obturation.

Obturation

- The contemporary method of obturating an open apex involves the utilisation of mineral trioxide aggregate (MTA) cement or a bioceramic cement (Gaitonde and Bishop 2007).
- Various devices are available to transport the MTA to the apex (Figure 26.5).
- MTA is packed sequentially down the canal utilising a variety of endodontic pluggers to create a block of material at least 4 mm in length at the apex (Figure 26.6).
- Once 4 mm of the apical portion of the canal is completed, the remaining walls of the canal should be cleansed of any MTA, and thermoplastic GP with sealer is placed to 3 mm below the CEJ and a definitive coronal restoration (Figure 26.7).

KEY POINTS

- Trauma can cause the cessation of root development resulting in a tooth with thin dentinal walls, an open apex, and a periapical lesion.
- An open apex presents with different canal preparation and obturation challenges due to the large size of both the canal and the apex.
- MTA and bioceramics can allow for more optimal treatment than traditional rubber-based obturation.
- These teeth are inherently weak and may develop root fracture.

27 Root resorption – external replacement

Figure 27.1 Periapical radiograph of a maxillary right incisor that was (a) intruded and (b) subsequently developed replacement resorption. Note the missing periodontal ligament space, poorly defined root outline and no radiolucency with the root appearing to have a trabecular pattern.

(a)   (b)

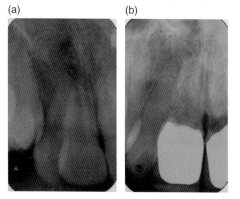

Figure 27.2 (a) Clinical appearance of an infra occluded maxillary left central incisor that has resisted orthodontic forces due to replacement resorption after dental trauma. (b) The periapical radiograph showing extensive replacement and invasive cervical resorption.

(a)   (b)

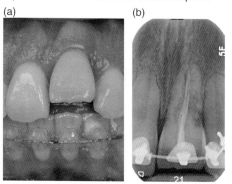

Figure 27.3 (a and b) Periapical radiographs of maxillary right central and left lateral incisors that have historical endodontic treatments that have had no effect on the replacement resorption. Note the left lateral incisor root has almost completely been replaced with bone, this is advantageous when considering future implant options. (c) Clinical appearance of the resorbed teeth. Key features to note: the historical enamel-dentine fracture of the maxillary right incisor, reduced mesio-distal prosthetic space of the missing left central incisor and the significant gingival zenith discrepancy.

(a)   (b)   (c)

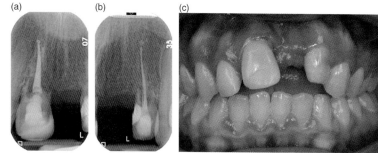

Figure 27.4 (a) Clinical appearance of a maxillary left central incisor with a history of trauma that developed replacement resorption and has infra-occluded. Note the discrepancy of the gingival zeniths. As the patients age is beyond the point of significant alveolar growth, further infra-occluded is unlikely and the incisal edge can be levelled with composite resin. (b) Final result, note the favourable low smile line hiding the gingival asymmetry.

(a)

(b)

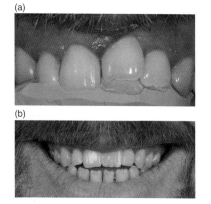

Figure 27.5 (a) Clinical appearance of a previously injured maxillary right central incisor in a growing patient that has significantly infra-occluded due to replacement resorption. Note, the adjacent incisors have tipped into the prosthetic space and the significant vertical hard and soft tissue discrepancy. (b) Clinical appearance of the central incisor decoronated to the level of the CEJ to preserve hard and soft tissue. This treatment should have been delivered much sooner to avoid such a sizeable vertical hard and soft tissue defect that will make definitive prosthodontics much more challenging.

(a)

(b)

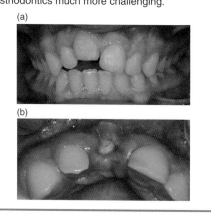

Dental Trauma at a Glance, First Edition. Aws Alani and Gareth Calvert. © 2021 John Wiley & Sons Ltd. Published 2021 by John Wiley & Sons Ltd.
Companion website: www.wiley.com/go/alani/dental_trauma

Definition

External replacement root resorption is the replacement of periodontal ligament, cementum and root dentine by alveolar bone (Figure 27.1).

Aetiology

The resorptive process occurs when there has been damage and subsequent necrosis of the periodontal ligament. Most commonly, this is due to luxation and avulsion injuries. Osteoclasts resorb exposed root dentine, which is replaced with alveolar bone by osteoblasts. The resorption usually continues until the entire root has been replaced by bone.

Prevalence

Approximately 30–60% of luxation and avulsion injuries at 10 years have signs of external replacement root resorption. The time after the injury and the rate of progression of the replacement resorption is impossible to quantify without follow-up (Andreasen & Andreasen 1992).

Clinical examination

- External replacement root resorption is commonly asymptomatic.
- The clinical crown of the affected tooth appears normal.
- Percussion of the tooth will reveal a high-pitched tone or metallic sound.
- There will be no physiological mobility.
- There maybe asymmetry of the gingival zenith points.
- The incisal level of the tooth may be more apical in position when compared to the adjacent teeth; this is infra-occlusion, also known as ankylosis.

Pulp test findings

As the resorption occurs on the external root surface, the pulp is unaffected and should respond positively.

Radiographic findings

Two periapical radiographs from different angles are recommended.

There will be no obvious periodontal ligament space.

The root outline is not well defined.

The parallel lines of the root canal system will be intact.

The resorption is not radiolucent as the root is being replaced by bone, so the resorptive area will appear with a trabecular pattern.

The resorption can appear at any position along the root surface.

There is commonly no periapical radiolucency.

Additional imaging such as a small field of view cone beam CT can be useful to examine the extent of the resorption.

Implications

There is no treatment modality that will cease the replacement resorption process.

If more than 20% of the root surface has undergone external replacement root resorption, the tooth will lose its physiological mobility and will not be moved by orthodontic forces (Figure 27.2).

The resorption will continue in spite of endodontic treatment (Figure 27.3).

A growing patient should be monitored regularly for signs of infra-occlusion so that early management can be instigated if required.

Management

As there is no effective management to cease external replacement root resorption, the affected tooth can be monitored until such time as the following occur (Cohenca and Stabholz 2007):

1 *Infra-occlusion of less than 2mm.* Composite resin can be applied to the incisal edge of the affected tooth to improve the aesthetics (Figure 27.4).
2 *Infra-occlusion of 2mm or more.* The risk of developing a severe vertical hard and soft tissue defect that will compromise prosthetic replacement of the injured tooth later in life is now significant.

Therefore, decoronation below the cemento-enamel junction of the crown and prosthetic replacement should be carried out. This will allow normal development of the adjacent supporting tissues and the adjacent teeth not to tip into the space (Figure 27.5).
3 *Symptoms.* The affected tooth should be extracted, and prosthetic replacement considered.
4 *Fracture.* The affected tooth can be decoronated or completely extracted depending on the situation, and prosthetic replacement considered.

Follow-up

Clinical and radiographic review on an annual basis or more regularly as per the original trauma injury follow-up.

Prognosis

If the external replacement root resorption is progressive, alternative tooth replacement options are inevitable.

Key Points

- External replacement root resorption is the replacement of root structure by bone progressing from the external surface of the root inward.
- Radiographically, the parallel lines of the root canal walls will be intact, but the periodontal ligament space will be missing.
- There is no physiological mobility, and a high-pitched note on percussion.
- Endodontic therapy will not cease the resorption process.
- If infra-occlusion occurs by 2mm or more, a coronectomy should be considered.

28 Root resorption – external cervical

Figure 28.1 Variations in clinical appearance of external cervical resorption. (a) Large lesion of maxillary left canine, obvious pink spot discolouration in the crown and breach of the labial enamel. (b) Gingival erythema and oedema associated with enamel defect labial of the maxillary left central incisor. (c) Palatal view of enamel breakdown and gingival tissue ingrowth into the palatal cavity of the maxillary right central incisor. (d) Early lesion with small enamel defect and gingival erythema of the maxillary right central incisor, (e) magnified image showing the vascular nature and invasion into the dental hard tissue.

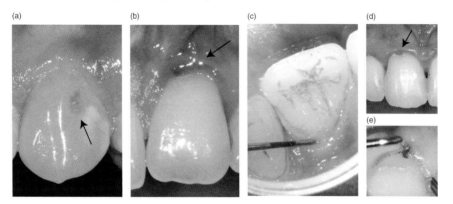

Figure 28.2 Illustration describing the radiographic appearance of external cervical resorption superimposed on the pulp canal outline

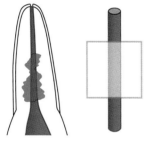

Figure 28.3 Radiographic appearance of various external cervical resorption lesions. (a) A large well defined lesion of the maxillary left lateral incisor, beginning on the mesial aspect and expanding symmetrically from the CEJ, note the parallel lines of the pulp canal are still visible and there is no periapical radiolucency. (b) Smaller resorption lesion affecting the maxillary right canine, again note parallel lines of the pulp canal are still visible and there is no periapical radiolucency. (c) A much more diffuse and extensive pattern of external cervical resoprtion affecting the maxillary left canine. (d) Sagital slice of a CBCT showing the resorption on the palatal aspect extending toward the pulp at the level of the CEJ. (e) Axial slice of a CBCT showing resorption of both the maxillary left central and right lateral incisors. Note the pulp has been clearly breached by the resorption on the lateral incisor.

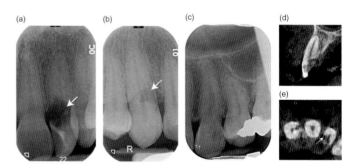

Figure 28.4 Clinical appearance of (a) external cervical root resorption under magnification after elevating a mucoperiosteal flap, note the two areas of enamel breakdown and invasion of the soft tissue, (b) the resorption lesion has been mechanically and chemically debrided, note the pre dentine layer still intact protecting the pulp, (c) the cavity has been restored and polished, note the haemostasis and sound margin of apical dentine.

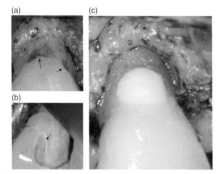

Figure 28.5 (a) Clinical appearance of a maxillary right central incisor decoronated due to the cervical resorption on the mesial surface, note the vascular nature of the lesion. (b) Clinical appearance of an extracted maxillary incisor due to extensive cervical resorption, note the undermined dental hard tissue and intact soft tissue lesion.

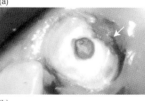
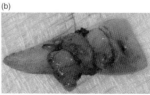

Dental Trauma at a Glance, First Edition. Aws Alani and Gareth Calvert. © 2021 John Wiley & Sons Ltd. Published 2021 by John Wiley & Sons Ltd.
Companion website: www.wiley.com/go/alani/dental_trauma

Definition

External cervical root resorption is the destruction of dental hard tissue by clastic cells on the external root surface at the cervical region.

Aetiology

While the exact aetiology of external cervical resorption is not known, the resorptive process occurs when there has been damage to the periodontal ligament and subepithelial cementum layer. Therefore, osteoclastic cells from the adjacent periodontium settle on the exposed root dentine and begin the resorption process. The fibrovascular resorption lesion may undergo osseous repair in rare circumstances, but most commonly, the resorptive lesion will progress to invade the root dentine.

Prevalence

External cervical resorption prevalence is rare in the general population. However, approximately 30% of cases have a history of dental trauma (Heithersay 1999). Dental trauma injuries that include damage to the periodontal ligament, including lateral luxation, avulsion, and intrusion injuries, are most commonly associated with external cervical root resorption. The most commonly identified tooth is the maxillary incisor.

Clinical examination

- In the early stages, external cervical root resorption is asymptomatic.
- However, the patient may present with symptoms of pulpitis or dentine hypersensitivity.
- Once the resorptive lesion is extensive, pink discolouration to the clinical crown can be observed (Figure 28.1).
- There can be a discrete periodontal pocket into the resorption defect or an obvious ingrowth of soft tissue with loss of tooth structure (Figure 28.1).
- When probed, the root surface will be firm, unlike a carious lesion. The lesion will then usually display copious bleeding due to its vascular nature (Figure 28.1).

Pulp test findings

As the resorption occurs on the external root surface, the pulp is unaffected and should respond positively.

If the resorptive lesion is extensive and breaches the root canal system, only then may the pulp become necrotic.

Radiographic findings

Two periapical radiographs from different angles are recommended.

As the radiolucent lesion is on the external root surface, it will appear to change position between the two angles. Therefore, it can be determined if the lesion is buccal or palatal.

The parallel lines of the root canal system will be intact (Figure 28.2).

The radiolucency will most commonly be at the cervical region. The radiolucency is not always well defined and appears superimposed on the root canal system (Figure 28.3).

The radiolucency can spread circumferentially around the pulp and also vertically in a coronal and apical direction.

There may or may not be a periapical radiolucency.

Additional imaging, such as a small field of view cone beam CT, can be useful to examine the extent of the circumferential spread and portal of entry (Figure 28.3).

Implications

When repositioning injured teeth, care must be taken not to further damage any portion of the cervical root surface, which may further promote external cervical root resorption.

If repositioning teeth with forceps, use gauze and grasp the crown of the injured tooth.

External cervical resorption can be misdiagnosed as caries and internal resorption.

Management options

The management of external cervical root resorption is much easier when detected early and can benefit from endodontic specialist input.

The exact location of the resorptive lesion must be identified. If there are no signs of hard tissue repair, the following options are available:

1 If accessible and amenable to repair, a mucoperiosteal flap is raised. The resorptive lesion and a rim of sound root surface is exposed. The resorptive lesion is then mechanically and chemically debrided.

The cavity can be restored with a material that is not sensitive to moisture, fast setting, and easily adjusted (Figure 28.4).

The mucoperiosteal flap is repositioned.

If the root canal system is breached during this procedure, orthograde endodontic therapy should be completed.

2 If from the pre-operative cone beam CT imaging, there is an obvious pulp breach by the external cervical root resorption, orthograde endodontic treatment can be initiated before surgical repair.

3 Alternatively, if the resorptive lesion is inaccessible or extensive, the tooth can be monitored in the medium to long term. The patient should be made aware that the tooth is likely to require further treatment in the future such as decoronation or extraction and prosthetic replacement (Figure 28.5).

Follow up

Clinical and radiographic review on an annual basis for up to four years or more regularly as per the original trauma injury follow up.

Prognosis

The earlier the detection and smaller the lesion, the better the prognosis, though there is no good quality long term outcome data.

> **KEY POINTS**
> - External cervical root resorption has a variety of notable features.
> - Radiographically, the parallel lines of the root canal walls will be intact. The radiolucent expansion is superimposed on the root canal system.
> - A surgical approach to debride the lesion is the primary method of treatment.
> - The pulp is commonly vital; therefore, orthograde endodontic treatment will usually have no effect on the resorption process.

Root resorption – internal inflammatory

29

Figure 29.1 (a) This crowned maxillary right central incisor revealed the presence of internal inflammatory root resorption at a routine examination. (b) Periapical radiograph of the maxillary right central incisor showing a uniform symmetrical expansion of the pulp canal in the middle third, note the loss of the parallel lines of the root canal system and the normal periapical tissue. (c) Post operative periapical radiograph of maxillary right central incisor having been endodontically treated with revision of the extra coronal restoration.

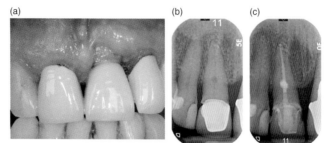

Figure 29.2 (a) Clinically normal appearance of the maxillary left central incisor incidentally noted to have internal inflammatory resorption. (b) Periapical radiograph of the maxillary left central incisor showing a uniform expansion of the pulp canal in the apical third, note the loss of the parallel lines of the root canal system and the presence of a periapical radiolucency. (c) Post operative periapical radiograph of maxillary left central incisor having been endodontically treated.

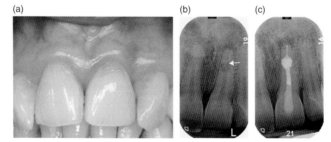

Figure 29.3 (a) Clinically normal appearance of the mandibular central incisors incidentally noted both to have internal inflammatory resorption. (b) Periapical radiograph of the mandibular central incisors showing a uniform expansion of the pulp canal in the middle and apical third, note the loss of the parallel lines of the root canal system, the periapical radiolucency associated with the right central incisor but not the left central incisor. (c) Post operative periapical radiograph of the mandibular central incisors following endodontic treatment, note the resolution of the periapical radiolucency.

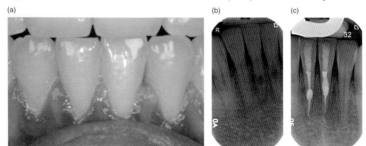

Figure 29.4 Clinical appearance of (a) the necrotic coronal pulp tissue, (b) the vital resorptive tissue being flushed out, (c) an intervisit medicament being placed inside the resorptive defect, (d) the contrast between the coronal irregular mottled canal dentine surface and the intact apical canal dentine (e) plugging the heated obturation material into the resorptive defect.

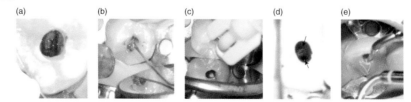

Dental Trauma at a Glance, First Edition. Aws Alani and Gareth Calvert. © 2021 John Wiley & Sons Ltd. Published 2021 by John Wiley & Sons Ltd.
Companion website: www.wiley.com/go/alani/dental_trauma

Definition

Internal inflammatory root resorption is the destruction of dental hard tissue from the internal surface of the root canal system by clastic cells within an inflammatory lesion.

Aetiology

The unmineralized layer of predentine usually protects the internal surface of the root canal dentine from clastic cells. However, after physical, chemical, or bacterial trauma to the predentine layer, multinucleated odontoclast cells may attach to the root canal dentine. If this is associated with inflammation, the dentine of the root canal system will be irreversibly damaged.

The pulp tissue coronal to the expanding lesion is necrotic. Conversely, the apical pulp, including the resorptive lesion, is usually vital, albeit inflamed. Therefore, the lesion will continue to expand laterally until the apical tissue has necrosed, or there has been endodontic intervention.

Prevalence

Internal inflammatory resorption is rare in the general population of 0.01–1%. However, physical trauma is a risk factor. Internal inflammatory resorption can happen at any time after an episode of dental trauma.

Clinical examination

- In the early stages, internal inflammatory resorption is commonly an incidental finding (Figure 29.1).
- If the resorption is extensive, the patient may present with symptoms of pulpitis or periradicular periodontitis.

Pulp test findings

There may be a positive response due to the potential of vital pulp tissue apically, which is propagating the resorption expansion. A negative response could suggest the pulp is completely necrotic and so the resorptive lesion would cease to progress.

Radiographic findings

Two periapical radiographs from different angles are recommended.

As the radiolucent lesion expands from the centre of the root outward, it will not change position with the shift in beam angulation (Figure 29.1).

The parallel lines of the root canal system will be lost and a well-defined symmetrical radiolucent circular or oval ballooning of the canal space (Figure 29.2).

This can happen at any length along the root canal system (Figure 29.3).

There may or may not be a periapical radiolucency.

If the resorption is extensive, it may breach the root completely and be associated with a lateral radiolucency.

Additional cone beam CT imaging can be useful in these instances.

Implications

Internal inflammatory resorption is propagated by a partially vital pulp. Therefore unless root canal therapy is initiated, the resorption lesion will continue.

The greater the size of the resorptive lesion, the more compromised the structural integrity of the tooth is and the increased chance of a pathological lateral perforation.

Management options

1 Root canal therapy should be initiated as soon as possible, and a referral should be considered for specialist treatment.

Due to the inflammatory tissue and vital pulp, expect to find copious haemorrhage from the root canal system. Care must be taken not to confuse this with a lateral perforation as initially, an apex locator may not give a consistent reading.

Once the tissue is excised, the haemorrhage will cease. Visibility will improve, and an apex locator will be able to determine if indeed there is a perforation present.

If the resorptive lesion is apically positioned, it can be awkward to locate and access the narrower unaltered apical root canal system.

Due to the irregular internal shape of the root canal system, disinfection and obturation become more complicated. Adjunctive ultrasonic irrigation methods should be employed for debridement and disinfection of the altered canal anatomy. Furthermore, it is sensible to utilise an intervisit medicament.

To ensure 3D obturation of the resorptive lesion, warm vertical compaction is the method of choice (Figure 29.4).

2 If a perforation is suspected or indeed confirmed, mineral trioxide aggregate or similar bioceramic material should be used to repair it.

3 If the resorptive lesion is extensive and compromising the structural integrity of the root with additional complications such as a pathological perforation and bone loss, then consideration should be given to extraction and prosthetic replacement.

Follow up

Clinical and radiographic review on an annual basis for up to four years or more regularly as per the original trauma injury follow up.

Prognosis

As internal resorption is rare, there is no good quality long-term outcome data. Radiographic survival data is suggested between 89–90% in the medium-term.

KEY POINTS

- Take two radiographs from different angles, the resorptive lesion will stay central in the root canal.
- Radiographically, the parallel lines of the root canal walls will be lost with a well-defined symmetrical radiolucent expansion of the canal space.
- Root canal therapy is indicated to cease the resorption.

30 Tooth replacement options

Figure 30.1 (a) Clinical appearance of the traumatic loss of a maxillary right central incisor after orthodontic space closure. (b) Post operative view of composite resin augmentation of the maxillary anteriors.

Figure 30.2 (a) Extra oral view of reduced maxillary lip support due to the traumatic loss of multiple maxillary teeth. (b) Intra oral view illustrating hard and soft tissue defects in both the horizontal and vertical dimension and limited inter-occlusal space. (c) Sagittal cone beam CT slice with a radiographic stent showing the extremely limited hard tissue volume. (d) Clinical view of a cobalt-chrome denture replacing the hard and soft tissue.

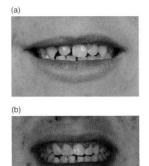

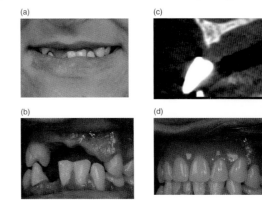

Figure 30.3 (a) Clinical appearance follow dental trauma to the maxillary incisors. (b) Post operative view of a resin retained bridge replacing the four maxillary incisors. Palatal view of the retainer wings on the maxillary canines (c) and (d).

Figure 30.4 (a) Clinical appearance of a narrow mandibular ridge subsequent to the traumatic loss of the four incisors. (b) Replacement of the 4 mandibular incisors with a conventional fixed-fixed bridge.

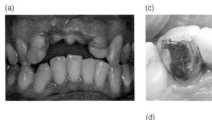

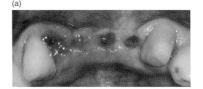

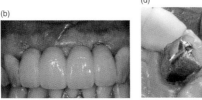

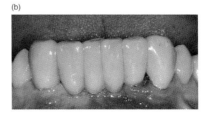

Figure 30.5 (a) Clinical appearance of a previously traumatised maxillary right central incisor that has discoloured and drifted. (b) Post operative clinical view after orthodontic alignment of the maxillary right central incisor. Clinical appearance of (c) an implant osteotomy site showing a deficient labial bony plate and (d) simultaneous grafting of the bony defect. (e) Post operative view of a single unit implant crown replacing the maxillary right central incisor.

Figure 30.6 Clinical appearance of donor sites (a) mandibular symphysis and (b) mandibular ramus for block bone grafting to furnish a recipient site with adequate bone volume to receive a dental implant.

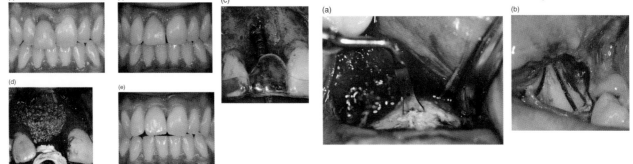

Dental Trauma at a Glance, First Edition. Aws Alani and Gareth Calvert. © 2021 John Wiley & Sons Ltd. Published 2021 by John Wiley & Sons Ltd.
Companion website: www.wiley.com/go/alani/dental_trauma

The prosthodontic management of tooth loss subsequent to trauma requires the assessment and management of various different factors (Alani et al. 2012). One important aspect to consider is the patient's plaque control and social factors, such as smoking, which will inevitably affect the longevity of both the teeth and associated prosthesis. Clinical factors include the bone stock within the edentate site, the restorative status of the adjacent teeth, the gingival biotype, and the occlusion. Another factor is the age of the patient. Patients in their early twenties or younger are more likely to undergo continued maxillary growth and, as such, are less likely to be ideal implant patients (Romanos et al. 2019). Wherever possible, the most minimally invasive treatment option should be considered from the outset. Resin-bonded bridges are an ideal consideration for patients who lack the requisite bone for implant placement or are too young (King et al. 2015).

Space closure

- If a tooth is lost, orthodontic space closure can be considered and assessed.
- This eliminates the lifelong maintenance of a prosthetic tooth replacement.
- However, this can have cosmetic shortcomings based on the feasibility of the adjacent teeth to be camouflaged with direct composite resin and or vital bleaching (Figure 30.1).

Factors to consider for a removable prosthesis

- Soft tissue support for the lip – necessitating a denture flange.
- Multiple missing teeth.
- Significant hard and soft tissue defects, particularly in a vertical dimension.
- Limited interocclusal space due to over eruption.
- Patient preference to avoid complex surgery.

Design considerations for a removable prosthesis

- Tooth supported wherever possible.
- Path of insertion.
- Indirect retention design.
- Maintenance of periodontal health.
- Replaces gingival tissue as well as tooth tissue for ideal tooth portions (Figure 30.2).
- Supports soft tissue profile.

Factors to consider for resin bonded bridge provision

- Periodontally healthy dentition.
- Unrestored abutment teeth with good surface area for bonding.
- Absence of severe parafunction.
- Interocclusal space and connector size.

Design features for resin bonded bridges-retainer wing

- Consistent 0.7 mm thickness in Nickel Chromium.
- Maximum palatal coverage and 180° engagement within the embrasure spaces.

- Consider abutment tooth preparation guide planes adjacent to the pontic site to improve bridge rigidity.
- 50 μm alumina sandblasted surface.

Design features for resin bonded bridges-pontic

- The ovate pontic is the most cleansable design (Figure 30.3).
- Light contact in the intercuspal position and absence of contact in lateral and anterior guidance.

Cementation

- Utilisation of an opaque cement is imperative.
- Rubber dam is required to ensure a moisture free field for adhesive cementation.
- Once fitted, the patient should be instructed in the use of floss and interproximal brushes.

Conventional fixed- fixed bridge

- The same basic principles of patient assessment should be adhered.
- The biological cost of tooth preparation and risk of endodontic intervention need consideration (Figure 30.4).

Factors to consider for implant placement

- The patient has completed maxillary growth.
- Periodontally healthy.
- There is adequate quality and quantity of bone (Figure 30.5), or there is the ability to graft the edentate site with adequate volume (Figure 30.6).
- Thick gingival biotype provides the best outcome.
- Vital structures such as the mental nerve and foramen, maxillary sinus and the floor of the nose are not close to the vicinity of the prospective implant site.
- The absence of risk factors such as periodontal disease, smoking, and poor oral hygiene.
- Static and dynamic occlusal relationships provide adequate space for the implant restoration.

Ongoing maintenance

- Patients need to be aware that tooth replacement prostheses require ongoing maintenance and review and will inevitably require replacement.
- 80% of resin-bonded bridges are expected to be present at 15 years, at which point they may or may not require replacement.
- At a conservative estimate, 1 in 3 implants may develop complications that may require intervention.

KEY POINTS

- Appreciate anterior tooth replacement is multifactorial.
- Realise that treatment planning should bear in mind the longevity of the treatment and future need for replacement.
- Provision of implant restorations need to take into account soft tissue and hard tissue factors as well as the age of the patient.
- Resin-bonded bridges require optimal adhesive technique for success.

31 Autotransplantation

Figure 31.1 Clinical appearance of (a) two premolars transplanted into the maxillary central incisor positions due to previous traumatic loss. (b) Orthodontic appliances to align the dentition and transplanted premolars. (c) Post orthodontic appearance of the transplanted premolars. (d) Composite additions to camouflage the transplanted premolars as maxillary central incisors, note the gingival asymmetry. Extra oral view (e) following orthodontic alignment and (f) following composite camouflage of the transplanted premolars as central incisors.

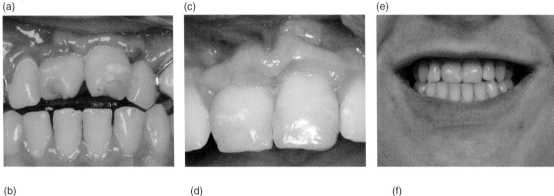

Figure 31.2 (a) Periapical radiograph of a transplanted premolar unit to the maxillary right central incisor position with a periapical radiolucency. Clinical appearance (b) extra orally and (c) of the transplanted premolar in the maxillary right central incisor position. (d) Clinical view of endodontic access to the transplanted premolar unit. Note the 90 degree rotation of the access cavity. (e) Post operative periapical radiograph of the endodontic treatment for the transplanted premolar unit.

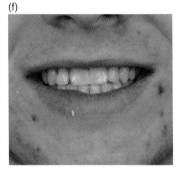

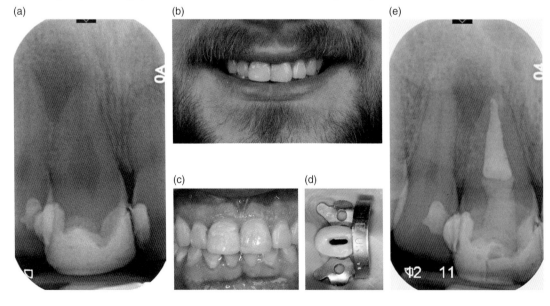

Definition

Autotransplantation is the replacement of a missing or unrestorable tooth by another immature donor tooth from the same patient.

Indication

Avulsion or a catastrophic injury to an incisor unit due to dental trauma in a growing, orthodontically amenable patient is an indication to consider autotransplantation.

Benefits

Interest in this procedure has been documented for some time because it has been shown to provide a natural physiologically adept option for the management of acquired tooth loss, maintenance of the alveolar bone and soft tissues and the avoidance of lifelong maintenance issues that may result from the provision of an implant or conventional prosthodontics.

Multidisciplinary team approach

There are a number of individual factors to consider regarding the recipient tooth site, the donor tooth site, remaining dentition, and prosthodontic alternatives. Therefore, an multidisciplinary approach is best suited to deliver this treatment.

The team should include specialists in
- Paediatric dentistry
- Orthodontics
- Oral surgery
- Restorative Dentistry

Assessment

The patient
- Medically fit and well.
- Treatment planned during active growth.
- Compliant with the prospect of complicated multi-faceted treatment.

Donor tooth
- Crown anatomy for an aesthetic outcome.
- Root anatomy can influence the complexity of surgery for atraumatic tooth removal and insertion into the recipient site.
- Stage of root development is key as an immature apex will more likely revascularise.
- These teeth are usually premolars as they help reduce potential crowding and may be extracted as part of an overall orthodontic plan.

Recipient site
- The prosthodontic envelope of the recipient site requires an assessment in terms of interocclusal space, mesiodistal space and the potential aesthetic outcome. These can be best appreciated through the fabrication of a wax up on mounted study casts simulating the proposed treatment.
- The surgical envelope needs to have the requisite bone volume to accommodate the donor tooth root. Cone beam CT is invaluable in assessing this aspect comprehensively.

Predictive factors

The key factor for long-term success is the healing of the periodontal ligament of the donor tooth.

Periodontal healing is significantly related to the stage of root development, surgical difficulty, and the recipient site alveolar bone (Kafourou et al. 2017).

The periodontal ligament can be damaged during mobilisation from the donor site, storage outside the mouth, and during placement into the recipient site. If the periodontal ligament is damaged beyond its capacity for repair, replacement resorption will occur, and the tooth will become infra-occluded, causing further unwanted complications (see Chapter 27).

Pulp revascularization is significantly related to the stage of root development (Kafourou et al. 2017). However, if the pulp does not revascularize following transplantation, endodontics may be required.

Unfavourable outcomes
- Pulp necrosis
- Lack of root development
- Replacement resorption
- Pulp canal obliteration
- Infection
- Failure

Maintenance of the autotransplanted tooth

Crown aesthetics
The donor tooth can be augmented with direct composite resin after it has been transplanted (Figure 31.1). Occasionally, the contralateral natural tooth may also require augmentation with composite resin to produce a symmetrical result.

Gingival aesthetics
The donor tooth is likely to develop asymmetrical gingival contour with the adjacent natural teeth. This is asssociated with the underlying root form and previous surgery. Surgical correction of the gingival symmetry is usually avoided unless absolutely critical and the patient has completed growth (Figure 31.1).

Endodontic therapy
Endodontic intervention may be required in the long term. Two important factors to consider are the 90° rotation of the tooth and augmentation of the crown, which makes conventional endodontic access more challenging (Figure 31.2).

KEY POINTS
- Autotransplantation is a predictable solution for the replacement of missing or unrestorable incisors in the growing patient (Akhlef et al. 2018; Rohof et al. 2018).
- Healing of the periodontal ligament is a critical factor.
- Endodontic treatment can be complicated by the donor premolar being rotated 90° and augmented with composite.

32 The role of orthodontics

Figure 32.1 (a) Pre and (b) post operative lateral views of a large overjet reduced by orthodontic therapy.

(a) 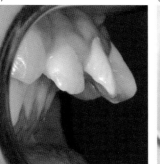   (b)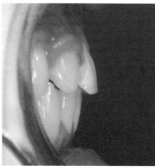

Figure 32.2 (a) Clinical appearance of a traumatically extruded maxillary central incisors. (b) Occlusal view showing a bonded palatal orthodontic retainer which has likely prevented the complete avulsion of the central incisors.

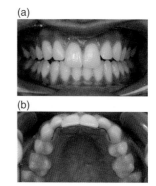

(a)

(b)

Figure 32.3 Periapical radiograph of intruded maxillary (a) right and (b) left central incisors with orthodontic appliances in-situ attempting to extrude the intruded incisors. Note the difference in incisal edge position of the central incisors, lack of complete periodontal ligament space and significant areas of root resorption. (c) Post operative clinical view of the camouflaged intruded maxillary central incisors as they were not able to be extruded.

(a)   (b)   (c)

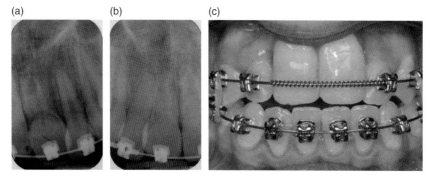

Figure 32.4 (a) Avulsion of the upper right central incisor without adequate repositioning of the luxated lateral incisor has resulted in a compromised prosthetic space. (b) Clinical view of a historic maxillary right central incisor avulsion and over time the adjacent teeth have drifted into the prosthetic space compromising pontic profile.

(a)

(b)

Figure 32.5 (a) Extra oral view of historic traumatic loss of the maxillary left central incisor, note the significant midline shift and asymmetry in the camouflaged teeth. (b) Intra oral view of space opening by orthodontics for a prosthetic replacement of the missing central incisor and correction of the midline shift. (c) Conventional preparation of the abutment teeth for a bridge. (d) Post operative extra oral view of the corrected midline and symmetry of the teeth and integration of the restorations.

(a)   (c)

(b)   (d)

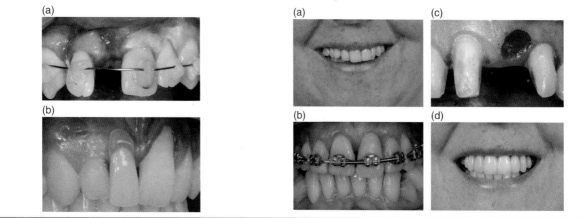

Dental Trauma at a Glance, First Edition. Aws Alani and Gareth Calvert. © 2021 John Wiley & Sons Ltd. Published 2021 by John Wiley & Sons Ltd.
Companion website: www.wiley.com/go/alani/dental_trauma

Managing dental trauma routinely requires a multidisciplinary approach. Having knowledge of all the potential treatment options will optimise a patient's journey and is the key to success.

Orthodontic treatment can be utilised in a number of ways and at various stages of a patient's journey to help prevent or manage dental trauma injuries.

Prevention of dental trauma

An increased overjet can triple the likelihood of experiencing dental trauma. Therefore the early identification and orthodontic management of a class II incisal relationship with a 6mm or more overjet could reduce that individual's risk (Glendor 2009) (Figure 32.1).

If the increased overjet is associated with incompetent lips (lip trap), orthodontic tooth movement to reduce the overjet could increase soft tissue protection of the maxillary dental hard tissues.

While there is limited high-level evidence in the literature, a bonded retainer for post orthodontic retention can have a protective influence on traumatised teeth. Figure 32.2 shows an extrusion injury of the maxillary central incisors; if the bonded retainer had not been in place, this could well have been an avulsion. Likewise, the resistance of the bonded retainer to luxation forces could minimise a tooth's displacement.

Immediate post dental trauma

Splinting

Round stainless steel orthodontic wire (0.016" or 0.4mm) is an ideal splint material as it is inexpensive, easy to manipulate, and passive.

Alternatively, if a tooth with a Twistflex wire-bonded retainer is damaged by dental trauma, the Twistflex wire is sometimes more easily tacked back together than fabricating a new splint.

Definitive treatment options

Orthodontic extrusion

Orthodontic alignment of mild intrusion injuries of up to 3mm that do not spontaneously re-erupt can be considered to reposition the traumatised tooth (Figure 32.3).

If the apical root portion of a crown-root fracture is deemed restorable by successful endodontic treatment, rapid orthodontic extrusion can gain more ferrule for a predicable restoration survival.

However, extruding the tooth in this manner is prone to a more buccally positioned root and requires high patient compliance.

Autotransplantation

For this treatment procedure to be successful, it requires the input of a number of dental specialities, ideally experienced in working in a team approach.

Orthodontic treatment to reposition adjacent teeth to the edentate site as well as managing buccal segment occlusion is key to the success of autotransplantation.

Space opening

Figure 32.4 shows a case of a central incisor avulsion and lateral luxation of the adjacent lateral incisor. Unfortunately, the luxated tooth has not been correctly repositioned. Therefore, orthodontics is required to recreate the prosthetic space for this edentate site. (Figure 32.5).

Teeth that infra-occlude allow the adjacent incisors to tip into the prosthetic space over time and growth of the patient. Orthodontics is required to optimise the mesiodistal dimension of the prosthetic space for a symmetrical definitive restoration (see Chapter 27).

Space closure

Alternatively, the space left by the loss of an incisor due to trauma can be closed. Composite augmentation and gingival surgery is usually required to camouflage the surrounding teeth to improve aesthetics (see Chapter 30).

There are a number of patient and tooth-related factors to consider for space opening versus space closure:

- Patient compliance and stage of development.
- Long-term maintenance of an artificial tooth replacement.
- Aesthetics.
- Orthodontic retention.

Risks associated with orthodontics

All orthodontic treatment is associated with root resorption; however, in the case of traumatised teeth, there is an additional risk. Orthodontic factors that may encourage resorption (Figure 32.3):

- Excessive forces
- Increased anchorage requirements
- Prolonged treatment times

However, for the overall treatment goals, these risks may have to be accepted as there maybe no reasonable alternative prosthodontic solution.

Long term orthodontic retention is still required

KEY POINTS
- Overjet reduction can reduce the risk of dental trauma.
- Orthodontic treatment can improve prosthetic outcomes for acquired tooth loss by optimising the edentate site.
- Orthodontic intervention has to be balanced with the increased risk of root resorption.

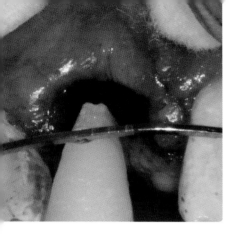

Appendix A: Splinting times and follow up intervals for fracture and displacement injuries in the adult dentition

Fracture injuries		Splint time	Follow-up intervals
	Infraction	NA	NA
	Enamel fracture	NA	Clinical and radiographic examination at 6 to 8 weeks initially and then at 1 year (If associated with a luxation injury, these review times should reflect the luxation)
	Enamel–dentine fracture	NA	Clinical and radiographic examination at 6 to 8 weeks initially and then at 1 year (If associated with a luxation injury, these review times should reflect the luxation)
	Enamel–dentine–pulp fracture	NA	Clinical and radiographic examination at 6 to 8 weeks, 3 months, 6 months, and then at 1 year (If associated with a luxation injury, these review times should reflect the luxation)
	Crown–root fracture with pulp exposure	NA	Clinical and radiographic examination at 1 week 6 to 8 weeks, 3 months, 6 months, and then annually for at least 5 years
	Crown–root fracture without pulp exposure	NA	Clinical and radiographic examination at 1 week, 6 to 8 weeks, 3 months, 6 months, and then annually for at least 5 years
	Root fracture Middle and apical root third Cervical root third	4 weeks 4 months	Clinical and radiographic examination at 4 weeks, 6 to 8 weeks, 4 months, 6 months, 1 year, and annually for at least 5 years
	Alveolar fracture	4 weeks	Clinical and radiographic examination at 4 weeks, 6 to 8 weeks, 4 months, 6 months, and annually for at least 5 years

Dental Trauma at a Glance, First Edition. Aws Alani and Gareth Calvert. © 2021 John Wiley & Sons Ltd. Published 2021 by John Wiley & Sons Ltd.
Companion website: www.wiley.com/go/alani/dental_trauma

Displacement injuries			Splint time	Follow-up intervals
	Concussion		NA	Clinical and radiographic examination 4 weeks, 1 year
	Subluxation		(If required 2 weeks)	Clinical and radiographic examination 2 weeks, 3 months, 6 months, 1 year
	Extrusive luxation		2 weeks	Clinical and radiographic examination 2 weeks, 4 weeks, 8 weeks, 3 months, 6 months, 1 year, annually for at least 5 years
	Lateral luxation		4 weeks	Clinical and radiographic examination 2 weeks, 4 weeks, 8 weeks, 3 months, 6 months, 1 year, annually for at least 5 years
	Intrusion Teeth with incomplete root formation Teeth with complete root formation repositioned		NA 4 weeks	Clinical and radiographic examination 2 weeks, 4 weeks, 8 weeks, 3 months, 6 months, 1 year, annually for at least 5 years
	Avulsion		2 weeks	Clinical and radiographic examination 2 weeks, 4 weeks, 3 months, 6 months, 1 year and annually for at least 5 years

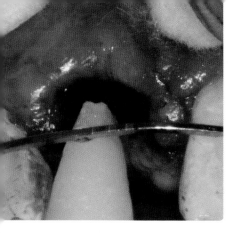

Appendix B: Management of dental trauma in the primary dentition

The management of certain injuries to the primary dentition differs from the permanent dentition and are outlined below. However, the same armamentarium, clinical examination, diagnosis, and treatment principles apply to both primary and permanent dentition, a description can be found in the relevant chapters.

'Fracture injuries'	Diagnosis	Treatment	Follow-up	Implications
Infraction	See Chapter 5	No treatment is necessary Post-operative instructions	No follow-up is required.	Eliminate the possibility of any concomitant injury.
Enamel fracture	See Chapter 6	Smooth sharp edges Post-operative instructions	No follow-up is required.	Eliminate the possibility of any concomitant injury.
Enamel dentine fracture	See Chapter 7	Restore all exposed dentine with either composite resin or glass ionomer Post-operative instructions	6 to 8 weeks	Eliminate the possibility of any concomitant injury.
Enamel dentine pulp fracture	See Chapter 8	Options can include: • Direct pulp capping • Partial 2 mm pulpotomy • Extraction Post-operative instructions	1 week 6 to 8 weeks 1 year	If compliance of the patient hinders proper pulp management, extraction is recommended.
Crown root fracture	See Chapter 9	Options can include: • Fragment removal and restore exposed dentine • Extraction in all other circumstances Post-operative instructions	1 week 6 to 8 weeks 1 year	If periradicular disease develops, the tooth may be extracted.
Crown root fracture with pulp involvement	See Chapter 10	Options can include: • Fragment removal, pulpotomy or root canal treatment and restore exposed dentine • Extraction in all other circumstances Post-operative instructions	1 week 6 to 8 weeks 1 year	If compliance of the patient hinders treatment or if periradicular disease develops, the tooth may be extracted.

Root fracture	See Chapter 11	Options include:
		• Non-displaced coronal fragment – accept
		• Displaced coronal fragment –
		  • Reposition and splint for four weeks
		  • Extract only the coronal fragment, leave the apical fragment to resorb
		Post-operative instructions
			1 week
			(4 weeks to remove splint if required)
			6 to 8 weeks
			1 year
			Annually until exfoliation
				If compliance of the patient hinders repositioning, extraction is recommended. Do not attempt to remove the fractured apical portion as this may injure the successor's development. If periradicular disease develops, the tooth may be extracted.

Alveolar fracture	See Chapter 12	Reposition the displaced segment Splint for four weeks Post-operative instructions	1 week 4 weeks (splint removal) 8 weeks 1 year 6 years of age	General anaesthesia may be required. If unfavourable healing, such as periradicular disease becomes evident, a referral should be made to a paediatric dentistry unit.

Dental Trauma at a Glance, First Edition. Aws Alani and Gareth Calvert. © 2021 John Wiley & Sons Ltd. Published 2021 by John Wiley & Sons Ltd.
Companion website: www.wiley.com/go/alani/dental_trauma

'Displacement injuries'	Diagnosis	Treatment	Follow-up	Implications
Concussion	See Chapter 13	No treatment is necessary Post-operative instructions	1 week 6 to 8 weeks	Eliminate the possibility of any concomitant injury.
Subluxation	See Chapter 14	No treatment is necessary Post-operative instructions	1 week 6 to 8 weeks	Eliminate the possibility of any concomitant injury.
Extrusion	See Chapter 15	Options: Treatment will depend on the degree of displacement, mobility, occlusion, and the patient's compliance: * Left to spontaneous align if no occlusal interference * Extraction in all other circumstances Post-operative instructions	1 week 6 to 8 weeks 1 year	If the primary tooth root is fully formed, extraction should be considered to prevent damage to the successor's development.
Intrusion	See Chapter 16	Options: * Spontaneous alignment (will take between 6 and 12 months) * Rapid referral to a paediatric dentistry unit Post-operative instructions	1 week 6 to 8 weeks 6 months 1 year 6 years of age	The risk of damage to the permanent successor should be mitigated at all costs.
Lateral luxation	See Chapter 17	Options: * Spontaneous repositioning if there is no occlusal disturbance (will occur in six months) * Repositioning when there is a mild occlusal interference and splint for four weeks * Extraction for teeth with severe displacement or there is a risk of ingestion/aspiration Post-operative instructions	1 week 4 weeks (splint removal) 8 weeks 6 months 1 year	If the primary tooth crown is displaced labially, the root will be displaced palatally toward the developing successor.
Avulsion	See Chapter 19	Do not replant the primary tooth If there is a primary tooth unaccounted for, radiographic examination should exclude a complete intrusion or displacement into the soft tissue Post-operative instructions	6 to 8 weeks 6 years of age	The risk of damage to the permanent successor outweighs the benefit of replantation.

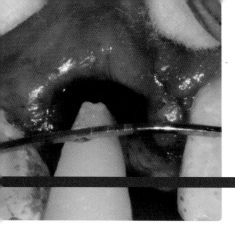

References

Chapter 1

Glendor, U. (2009). Aetiology and risk factors related to traumatic dental injuries-a review of the literature. *Dental Traumatology* 25 (1): 19–31.

Chapter 2

Benson, B.W., Mohatadi, N.G., Rose, M.S., and Meeuwisse, W.H. (1999). Head and neck injuries among ice hockey players wearing full face shields vs half face shields. *Journal of the American Medical Association* 282: 2328–2332.

Fernandes, L.M., Neto, J.C.L., Lima, T.F.R. et al. (2019). The use of mouthguards and prevalence of dento-alveolar trauma among athletes: a systematic review and meta-analysis. *Dental Traumatology* 35 (1): 54–72.

Johnston, T. and Messer, L.B. (1996). An in vitro study of the efficacy of mouthguard protection for dentoalveolar injuries in deciduous and mixed dentitions. *Endodontics & Dental Traumatology* 12: 277–285.

Kelly, P., Sanson, T., Strange, G., and Orsay, E. (1991). A prospective study of the impact of helmet usage on motorcycle trauma. *Annals of Emergency Medicine* 20: 852–856.

Reath, D.B., Kirby, J., Lynch, M., and Maull, K.I. (1989). Patterns of maxillofacial injuries in restrained and unrestrained motor vehicle crash victims. *The Journal of Trauma* 29: 806–809.

Chapter 3

Chauhan, R., Rasaratnam, L., Alani, A., and Djemal, S. (2016). Adult dental trauma: what should the dental practitioner know? *Primary Dental Journal* 5 (3): 70–81.

Djemal, S. and Singh, P. (2016). Smartphones and dental trauma: the current availability of apps for managing traumatic dental injuries. *Dental Traumatology* 32 (1): 52–57.

Chapter 4

Bastos, J.V., Goulart, E.M., and de Souza Côrtes, M.I. (2014). Pulpal response to sensibility tests after traumatic dental injuries in permanent teeth. *Dental Traumatology* 30 (3): 188–192.

Bourguignon, C., Cohenca, N., Lauridsen, E. et al. (2020). International association of dental traumatology guidelines for the management of traumatic dental injuries: 1. Fractures and luxations. *Dental Traumatology* https://doi.org/10.1111/edt.12578. Advance online publication.

Chapter 5

Andreasen, F.M., Vestergaard, B., and Pedersen, B. (1985). Prognosis of luxated permanent teeth – the development of pulp necrosis. *Endodontics & Dental Traumatology* 1 (5): 207–220.

Chapter 6

Andreasen, J.O. (1970). Etiology and pathogenesis of traumatic dental injuries. A clinical study of 1,298 cases. *Scandinavian Journal of Dental Research* 78 (7): 329–342.

Andreasen, F.M., Vestergaard, B., and Pedersen, B. (1985). Prognosis of luxated permanent teeth – the development of pulp necrosis. *Endodontics & Dental Traumatology* 1 (5): 207–220.

Andreasen, F.M., Noren, J.G., Andreasen, J.O. et al. (1995). Long-term survival of crown fragment bonding in the treatment of crown fractures. A multi-center clinical study of fragment retention. *Quintessence International* 26 (4): 669–681.

Gutz, D.P. (1971). Fractured permanent incisors in a clinic population. *ASDC Journal of Dentistry for Children* 38 (2): 94–121.

Lauridsen, E., Hermann, N.V., Gerds, T.A. et al. (2012). Combination injuries 3. The risk of pulp necrosis in permanent teeth extrusion or lateral luxation and concomitant crown fractures without pulp exposure. *Dental Traumatology* 28 (2): 379–385.

Rauschenberger, C.R. and Hovland, E.J. (1995). Clinical management of crown fractures. *Dental Clinics of North America* 39 (8): 25–51.

Ravn, J.J. (1981). Follow-up study of permanent incisors with enamel cracks as a result of an acute trauma. *Scandinavian Journal of Dental Research* 89: 117–123.

Robertson, A. (1998). A retrospective evaluation of patients with uncomplicated crown fractures and luxation injuries. *Endodontics & Dental Traumatology* 14 (6): 245–256.

Stalhane, I. and Hedegard, B. (1975). Traumatized permanent teeth in children aged 7–15 years. Part II. *Swedish Dental Journal* 68 (1): 157–169.

Chapter 7

Andreasen, J.O. (1970). Etiology and pathogenesis of traumatic dental injuries. A clinical study of 1,298 cases. *Scandinavian Journal of Dental Research* 78 (7): 329–342.

Andreasen, F.M., Vestergaard, B., and Pedersen, B. (1985). Prognosis of luxated permanent teeth – the development of pulp necrosis. *Endodontics & Dental Traumatology* 1 (5): 207–220.

Andreasen, F.M., Noren, J.G., Andreasen, J.O. et al. (1995). Long-term survival of crown fragment bonding in the treatment of crown fractures. A multi-center clinical study of fragment retention. *Quintessence International* 26 (4): 669–681.

Gutz, D.P. (1971). Fractured permanent incisors in a clinic population. *ASDC Journal of Dentistry for Children* 38 (2): 94–121.

Hedegard, B. (1975). Traumatized permanent teeth in children aged 7–15 years. Part II. *Swedish Dental Journal* 68 (8): 157–169.

Lauridsen, E., Hermann, N.V., Gerds, T.A. et al. (2012). Combination injuries 3. The risk of pulp necrosis in permanent teeth extrusion or lateral luxation and concomitant crown fractures without pulp exposure. *Dental Traumatology* 28 (2): 379–385.

Rauschenberger, C.R. and Hovland, E.J. (1995). Clinical management of crown fractures. *Dental Clinics of North America* 39 (8): 25–51.

Dental Trauma at a Glance, First Edition. Aws Alani and Gareth Calvert. © 2021 John Wiley & Sons Ltd. Published 2021 by John Wiley & Sons Ltd.
Companion website: www.wiley.com/go/alani/dental_trauma

Robertson, A. (1998). A retrospective evaluation of patients with uncomplicated crown fractures and luxation injuries. *Endodontics & Dental Traumatology* 14 (6): 245–256.

Stalhane Olsburgh, S., Jacoby, T., and Krejci, I. (2002). Crown fractures in the permanent dentition: pulpal and restorative considerations. *Dental Traumatology* 18 (6): 103–115.

Chapter 8

Andreasen, J.O. (1970). Etiology and pathogenesis of traumatic dental injuries. A clinical study of 1,298 cases. *Scandinavian Journal of Dental Research* 78 (7): 329–342.

Andreasen, J.O. and Andreasen, F.M. (eds.) (1993). Crown fractures. In: *Textbook and Color Atlas of Traumatic Injuries to the Teeth*, 3e, 280–304. Copenhagen: Blackwell Munksgaard.

Bakland, L.K. (2009). Revisiting traumatic pulpal exposure: materials, management principles and techniques. *Dental Clinics of North America* 13 (4): 661–673.

Bakland, L.K. and Andreasen, J.O. (2002). Will mineral trioxide aggregate replace calcium hydroxide in treating pulpal and periodontal healing complications subsequent to dental trauma. A review. *Dental Traumatology* 16 (1): 25–32.

Cvek, M. (1993). Partial pulpotomy in crown-fractures incisors – results 3 to 15 years after treatment. *Acta Stomatologica Croatica* 27 (5): 167–173.

Gutz, D.P. (1971). Fractured permanent incisors in a clinic population. *ASDC Journal of Dentistry for Children* 38 (2): 94–121.

Olsburgh, S., Jacoby, T., and Krejci, I. (2002). Crown fractures in the permanent dentition: pulpal and restorative considerations. *Dental Traumatology* 12 (3): 103–115.

Stalhane Olsburgh, S., Jacoby, T., and Krejci, I. (2002). Crown fractures in the permanent dentition: pulpal and restorative considerations. *Dental Traumatology* 18 (6): 103–115.

Chapter 9

Castro, J.C., Poi, W.R., Manfrin, T.M., and Zina, L.G. (2005). Analysis of the crown fractures and crown-root fractures due to dental trauma assisted by the integrated clinic from 1992 to 2002. *Dental Traumatology* 21 (3): 121–126.

de Castro, M.A., Poi, W.R., de Castro, J.C. et al. (2010). Crown and crown-root fractures: an evaluation of the treatment plans for management proposed by 154 specialists in restorative dentistry. *Dental Traumatology* 26 (3): 236–242.

Elkhadem, A., Mickan, S., and Richards, D. (2014). Adverse events of surgical extrusion in treatment for crown-root and cervical root fractures: a systematic review of case series/reports. *Dental Traumatology* 30 (1): 1–14.

Chapter 10

Castro, J.C., Poi, W.R., Manfrin, T.M., and Zina, L.G. (2005). Analysis of the crown fractures and crown-root fractures due to dental trauma assisted by the integrated clinic from 1992 to 2002. *Dental Traumatology* 21 (3): 121–126.

de Castro, M.A., Poi, W.R., de Castro, J.C. et al. (2010). Crown and crown-root fractures: an evaluation of the treatment plans for management proposed by 154 specialists in restorative dentistry. *Dental Traumatology* 26 (3): 236–242.

Elkhadem, A., Mickan, S., and Richards, D. (2014). Adverse events of surgical extrusion in treatment for crown-root and cervical root fractures: a systematic review of case series/reports. *Dental Traumatology* 30 (1): 1–14.

Chapter 11

Andreasen, J.O., Andreasen, F.M., Mejàre, I., and Cvek, M. (2004). Healing of 400 intra-alveolar root fractures. 1. Effect of pre-injury and injury factors such as sex, age, stage of root development, fracture type, location of fracture and severity of dislocation. *Dental Traumatology* 20 (4): 192–202.

Andreasen, J.O., Ahrensburg, S.S., and Tsilingaridis, G. (2012). Root fractures: the influence of type of healing and location of fracture on tooth survival rates -an analysis of 492 cases. *Dental Traumatology* 28 (5): 404–409.

Cvek, M., Tsilingaridis, G., and Andreasen, J.O. (2008). Survival of 534 incisors after intra-alveolar root fracture inpatients aged 7–17 years. *Dental Traumatology* 24 (4): 379–387.

Majorana, A., Pasini, S., Bardellini, E., and Keller, E. (2002). Clinical and epidemiological study of traumatic root fractures. *Dental Traumatology* 18 (2): 77–80.

Chapter 12

Andreasen, J.O. and Lauridsen, E. (2015). Alveolar process fractures in the permanent dentition. Part 1. Etiology and clinical characteristics. A retrospective analysis of 299 cases involving 815 teeth. *Dental Traumatology* (6): 442–447.

Andreasen, J.O., Ahrensburg, S.S., Hillerup, S. et al. (2011). Alveolar fractures in the permanent dentition. Part 3. A clinical prospective study of 83 cases involving 197 teeth. Effect of treatment factors upon healing complications. *Dental Traumatology* (27): 698–672.

Lauridsen, E., Gerds, T., and Andreasen, J.O. (2016). Alveolar process fractures in the permanent dentition. Part 2. The risk of healing complications in teeth involved in an alveolar process fracture. *Dental Traumatology* 32: 128–139.

Chapter 13

Borum, M.K. and Andreasen, J.O. (2001). Therapeutic and economic implications of traumatic dental injuries in Denmark: an estimate based on 7549 patients treated at a major trauma centre. *International Journal of Paediatric Dentistry* 11 (4): 249–258.

Hermann, N.V., Lauridsen, E., Ahrensburg, S.S. et al. (2012). Periodontal healing complications following concussion and subluxation injuries in the permanent dentition: a longitudinal cohort study. *Dental Traumatology* 28 (5): 386–393.

Lauridsen, E., Hermann, N.V., Gerds, T.A. et al. (2012). Combination injuries 2. The risk of pulp necrosis in permanent teeth with subluxation injuries and concomitant crown fractures. *Dental Traumatology* 28 (5): 371–378.

Chapter 14

Borum, M.K. and Andreasen, J.O. (2001). Therapeutic and economic implications of traumatic dental injuries in Denmark: an estimate based on 7549 patients treated at a major trauma centre. *International Journal of Paediatric Dentistry* 11 (4): 249–258.

Hermann, N.V., Lauridsen, E., Ahrensburg, S.S. et al. (2012). Periodontal healing complications following concussion and subluxation injuries in the permanent dentition: a longitudinal cohort study. *Dental Traumatology* 28 (5): 386–393.

Lauridsen, E., Hermann, N.V., Gerds, T.A. et al. (2012). Combination injuries 2. The risk of pulp necrosis in permanent teeth with subluxation injuries and concomitant crown fractures. *Dental Traumatology* 28 (5): 371–378.

Chapter 15

Borum, M.K. and Andreasen, J.O. (2001). Therapeutic and economic implications of traumatic dental injuries in Denmark: an estimate based on 7549 patients treated at a major trauma centre. *International Journal of Paediatric Dentistry* 11 (4): 249–258.

Hermann, N.V., Lauridsen, E., Ahrensburg, S.S. et al. (2012). Periodontal healing complications following concussion and subluxation injuries in the permanent dentition: a longitudinal cohort study. *Dental Traumatology* 28 (5): 386–393.

Lauridsen, E., Hermann, N.V., Gerds, T.A. et al. (2012). Combination injuries 2. The risk of pulp necrosis in permanent teeth with subluxation injuries and concomitant crown fractures. *Dental Traumatology* 28 (5): 371–378.

Chapter 16

Andreasen, J.O., Bakland, L.K., Matras, R.C., and Andreasen, F.M. (2006a). Traumatic intrusion of permanent teeth. Part 1. An epidemiological study of 216 intruded permanent teeth. *Dental Traumatology* 22 (2): 83–92.

Andreasen, J.O., Bakland, L.K., and Andreasen, F.M. (2006b). Traumatic intrusion of permanent teeth. Part 2. A clinical study of the effect of preinjury and injury factors, such as sex, age, stage of root development, tooth location, and extent of injury including number of intruded teeth on 140 intruded permanent teeth. *Dental Traumatology* 22 (2): 90–98.

Wigen, T.I., Agnalt, R., and Jacobsen, I. (2008). Intrusive luxation of permanent incisors in Norwegians aged 6–17 years: a retrospective study of treatment and outcome. *Dental Traumatology* 24 (6): 612–618.

Chapter 17

Bastos, J.V., Goulart, E.M., and de Souza Côrtes, M.I. (2014). Pulpal response to sensibility tests after traumatic dental injuries in permanent teeth. *Dental Traumatology* 30 (3): 188–192.

Borum, M.K. and Andreasen, J.O. (2001). Therapeutic and economic implications of traumatic dental injuries in Denmark: an estimate based on 7549 patients treated at a major trauma centre. *International Journal of Paediatric Dentistry* 11 (4): 249–258.

Lauridsen, E., Hermann, N.V., Gerds, T.A. et al. (2012a). Combination injuries 1. The risk of pulp necrosis in permanent teeth with concussion injuries and concomitant crown fractures. *Dental Traumatology* 28 (5): 364–370.

Lauridsen, E., Hermann, N.V., Gerds, T.A. et al. (2012b). Combination injuries 2. The risk of pulp necrosis in permanent teeth with subluxation injuries and concomitant crown fractures. *Dental Traumatology* 28 (5): 371–378.

Lauridsen, E., Hermann, N.V., Gerds, T.A. et al. (2012c). Combination injuries 3. The risk of pulp necrosis in permanent teeth with extrusion or lateral luxation and concomitant crown fractures without pulp exposure. *Dental Traumatology* 28 (5): 379–385.

Chapter 19

Andersson, L., Andreasen, J.O., Day, P. et al. (2017). Guidelines for the management of traumatic dental injuries: 2. Avulsion of permanent teeth. *Pediatric Dentistry* 15 (6): 412–419.

De Brier, N., Dorien, O., Borra, V. et al. (2020). Storage of an avulsed tooth prior to replantation: a systematic review and meta-analysis. *Dental Traumatology* https://doi.org/10.1111/edt.12564. Advance online publication.

Fouad, A.F., Abbott, P.V., Tsilingaridis, G. et al. (2020). International association of dental traumatology guidelines for the management of traumatic dental injuries: 2. Avulsion of permanent teeth. *Dental Traumatology* https://doi.org/10.1111/edt.12573. Advance online publication.

Pohl, Y., Filippi, A., and Kirschner, H. (2005a). Results after replantation of avulsed permanent teeth. I. Endodontic considerations. *Dental Traumatology* 21 (2): 80–92.

Pohl, Y., Filippi, A., and Kirschner, H. (2005b). Results after replantation of avulsed permanent teeth. II. Periodontal healing and the role of physiologic storage and antiresorptive-regenerative therapy. *Dental Traumatology* 21 (2): 93–101.

Pohl, Y., Wahl, G., Filippi, A., and Kirschner, H. (2005c). Results after replantation of avulsed permanent teeth. III. Tooth loss and survival analysis. *Dental Traumatology* 21 (2): 102–110.

Chapter 20

Borssén, E., Källestål, C., and Holm, A.K. (2002). Treatment time of traumatic dental injuries in a cohort of 16-year-olds in northern Sweden. *Acta Odontologica Scandinavica* 60 (5): 265–270.

Borum, M.K. and Andreasen, J.O. (2001). Therapeutic and economic implications of traumatic dental injuries in Denmark: an estimate based on 7549 patients treated at a major trauma centre. *International Journal of Paediatric Dentistry* 11 (4): 249–258.

Wong, F.S. and Kolokotsa, K. (2004). The cost of treating children and adolescents with injuries to their permanent incisors at a dental hospital in the United Kingdom. *Dental Traumatology* 20 (6): 327–332.

Chapter 21

Bourguignon, C., Cohenca, N., Lauridsen, E. et al. (2020). International association of dental traumatology guidelines for the management of traumatic dental injuries: 1. Fractures and luxations. *Dental Traumatology* https://doi.org/10.1111/edt.12578. Advance online publication.

Levin, L., Day, P., Hicks, L. et al. (2020). International association of dental traumatology guidelines for the management of traumatic dental injuries: general introduction. *Dental Traumatology* https://doi.org/10.1111/edt.12574. Advance online publication.

Chapter 22

Mandel, U. and Viidik, A. (1989). Effect of splinting on the mechanical and histological properties of the healing periodontal ligament in the vervet monkey (Cercopithecus aethiops). *Archives of Oral Biology* 34 (3): 209–217.

Chapter 23

Chen, E. and Abbott, P.V. (2011). Evaluation of accuracy, reliability, and repeatability of five dental pulp tests. *Journal of Endodontia* 37 (12): 1619–1623.

Chapter 24

McCabe, P.S. and Dummer, P.M. (2012). Pulp canal obliteration: an endodontic diagnosis and treatment challenge. *International Endodontic Journal* 45 (2): 177–197.

Chapter 25

Krastl, G., Allgayer, N., Lenherr, P. et al. (2013). Tooth discoloration induced by endodontic materials: a literature review. *Dental Traumatology* 29: 2–72.

Malmgren, B. and Hübel, S. (2012). Transient discoloration of the coronal fragment in intra-alveolar root fractures. *Dental Traumatology* 28: 200–243.

Setien, V.J., Roshan, S., and Nelson, P.W. (2008). Clinical management of discolored teeth. *General Dentistry* (56): 294–300.

Sulieman, M.A. (2008). An overview of tooth-bleaching techniques: chemistry, safety and efficacy. *Periodontology* 2000 (48): 148–169.

Chapter 26

Gaitonde, P. and Bishop, K. (2007). Apexification with mineral trioxide aggregate: an overview of the material and technique. *The European Journal of Prosthodontics and Restorative Dentistry* 15 (1): 41–45.

Chapter 27

Anderson, L., Blomlöf, L., Lindskog, S. et al. (1984). Tooth ankylosis. Clinical, radiographic and histological assessments. *International Journal of Oral Surgery* 13: 423–431. 2.

Andreasen, J.O. and Andreasen, F.M. (1992). Root resorption following traumatic dental injuries. *Proceedings of the Finnish Dental Society* 88 (Suppl 1): 95–114.

Cohenca, N. and Stabholz, A. (2007). Decoronation -a conservative method to treat ankylosed teeth for preservation of alveolar ridge prior to permanent prosthetic reconstruction: literature review and case presentation. *Dental Traumatology* 23: 87–94.

Chapter 28

Heithersay, G.S. (1999). Invasive cervical resorption following trauma. *Australian Endodontic Journal* 25 (2): 79–85.

Chapter 30

Alani, A., Austin, R., and Djemal, S. (2012). Contemporary management of tooth replacement in the traumatized dentition. *Dental Traumatology* 28 (3): 183–192.

King, P.A., Foster, L.V., Yates, R.J. et al. (2015). Survival characteristics of 771 resin-retained bridges provided at a UK dental teaching hospital. *British Dental Journal* 218 (7): 423–428.

Romanos, G.E., Delgado-Ruiz, R., and Sculean, A. (2019). Concepts for prevention of complications in implant therapy. *Periodontology* 81 (1): 7–17.

Chapter 31

Akhlef, Y., Schwartz, O., Andreasen, J.O., and Jensen, S.S. (2018). Autotransplantation of teeth to the anterior maxilla: a systematic review of survival and success, aesthetic presentation and patient-reported outcome. *Dental Traumatology* 34: 20–27.

Kafourou, V., Tong, H.J., Day, P. et al. (2017). Outcomes and prognostic factors that influence the success of tooth autotransplantation in children and adolescents. *Dental Traumatology* 33: 393–399.

Rohof, E.C.M., Kerdijk, W., Jansma, J. et al. (2018). Autotransplantation of teeth with incomplete root formation: a systematic review and meta-analysis. *Clinical Oral Investigations* 22: 1613–1624.

Chapter 32

Glendor, U. (2009). Aetiology and risk factors related to traumatic dental injuries-a review of the literature. *Dental Traumatology* 25 (1): 19–31.

Index

Note: Page numbers in *italic* refer to figures.

Dental Trauma at a Glance, First Edition. Aws Alani and Gareth Calvert. © 2021 John Wiley & Sons Ltd. Published 2021 by John Wiley & Sons Ltd.
Companion website: www.wiley.com/go/alani/dental_trauma